A Book Series

Perfect At Last
WEIGHT

**An Evolutionary Perspective's Guide on
Attaining an Ideal Body Weight the Fastest,
Most Natural Way**

by Josephine Grace Chua Rojo, MD

Table of Contents

Copyright

First Printing: 2019

ISBN: 9781691732487

Unit 5B, 2nd Lacson St., Bacolod City, Negros Occidental, Philippines, 6100

www.healthandwellnessforless.info

Dedication

To my mother, *Julemar*, Tita Mama, *Angelie*, and husband *Uncle Jerome*, brothers, *Alvin, Andrew* and *Albert*, family and friends, who, in one way or another, appreciated my words enough to follow through and see the good results themselves. Without you, I wouldn't have the inspiration to start this.

Special thanks to my sister, *Jane Catherine*, for the unconditional love and support, not just in this book but in all days of my life.

Acknowledgement

Special thanks to *Kenneth Bryan*,
Marie Krielle Tasha and *Tyron Jon* for helping me in many other aspects necessary in producing this book.

About The Author

My name is Grace and I am a practicing medical doctor by profession. I took Bachelor of Arts in Psychology in college before I proceeded to medicine. The second I learned about how we evolved as humans, was the moment I developed both curiosity and fascination with how our body continuously responds like cavemen even to modern day challenges. Say for example, a traffic situation leaving one unable to do anything but be still. Such scenario triggers anxiety and sends modern men to resort to their *fight or flight response*. Thus, blood instinctively flows to hands and legs, in preparation to either engage in a physical fight or to run for one's life *(like how homo sapiens did it millions of years ago)*, making the legs restless for not being able to do anything, other than sit still and endure the traffic-induced pain. And as I went on, I realized that this holds true in almost any aspect of our day to day living, especially with our eating pattern.

We are in the 21st century but our body still functions the way it used to for the last thousands of years of its genetic existence. Like many of you, I have struggled with my weight for as long as I can remember. I have tried so many diet regimes but with no sustainable results. Growing up, I have always been on the heavier side. I am a 5-foot, 4.5 inches tall and the heaviest I have recorded weighing was 141 pounds.

Surely I have weighed more, but I just didn't have the courage to weigh myself during those times. I always look back to a transient time in high school and college where I considered to have been at my slimmest, most ideal body weight of 121 pounds. This may sound like it isn't a struggle since I never really reached the obese scale, but the truth is there is a real challenge in trying to lose weight when you are already within what is considered as "*normal*", but, non-ideal self.

My relationship with food is just something that I could not get a hold of. And it has deep roots since the same is a struggle with the rest of my family. Food has always been a source of comfort, happiness and part of every celebration. Skipping a meal is just out of the deal. Unintentional skipped meals are compensated immediately right after. But tragedy occurred in our family. The loss of my father and three of his other siblings in their early 50s consecutively for four years due to lifestyle disease, had me question my unhealthy habits and seriously thought about improving my overall wellness, starting with my weight.

And as I go back and see it in an *evolutionary perspective,* backed up by scientific evidence from my study of medicine, what I needed to do became clear. I did what nobody in my world thought I could ever do. And in a month's time, I achieved the body weight that I thought would only be in my dreams. From 140+ pounds, I became 115-118 and a BMI of 19-19.5. I always have the energy and the endurance to do my day to day tasks without difficulty that I used to have because of excess weight. With determination, adequate knowledge and proper mindset, your body weight can be perfect at last too

Disclaimer

The information written in this book is from the best of the author's knowledge with the sincerest intention to help. This book only intends to serve as a guide and does not intend to replace the specific medical advice given to each patient by his or her own physician. It will not substitute the medications currently prescribed to the reader for a specific illness. Any dietary and lifestyle recommendations mentioned in this book are wholly the personal view of the author. Readers are strongly advised to conduct their own research and consultations to verify the applicability of the texts written in this guide to each personal case. The author does not and will not derive any financial gain from organizations or companies mentioned in these texts. As of this writing, and as far as the knowledge of the author is concerned, there has been no medical emergency associated with the recommendations in this book. The reader is solely responsible for any lifestyle changes he or she may wish to proceed with after reading this book. It is strongly advised that consultation with your trusted physician should be done first prior to embarking on any lifestyle change especially for people with existing medical illness.

No copyright infringement is intended on the photos used in this book. Credits are given to the owners and sites where the photos were taken. Should there be any inadvertent copyright infringement committed, kindly contact the author so immediate rectification may be undertaken.

INTRODUCTION
Understanding Where We Came From

At least 700 million years ago, the closest ancestor of humans roamed the earth. They feed on whatever fresh fruits and vegetables available on their given location at that specific season. You see, once all the produce is consumed in that area, it might take some time before they can eat again. There will be days and even weeks of starvation and yet, they didn't die of hunger, they continued to live and persisted.

Fast-forward to 800,000 years ago, our more developed ancestors learned about controlled fire and eventually evolved to discover cooking. It allowed them to consume previously raw and inedible food sources which made them stronger, wiser and better. As hunters and gatherers, they can already eat meat and cook some variety of crops in addition to their previous diet. But despite this, still, there was no mode of food preservation at that point and whatever they got from days of hunting must be eaten in a short period of time to avoid spoilage. And what will follow are again prolonged days of hunger and no food at all, but they continued to live, until the next hunt is successful and everyone is once again fed.

Thus, if you try to imagine their normal day, breakfast aren't part of the usual deal, and dinner comes early since the danger of the night forces them to seek for a safe shelter away from predators, making their daily *window period of eating* very limited and far from our current timeframe of eating that is, eating whenever we are awake.

It's only about 10,000 B.C. that the transition from *hunter-gatherer stage* shifted to *stationary farming*. By this time, humans no longer need to travel places and hunt long distances just to eat. Instead, they can eat whenever crops and livestock are already set for harvest, signifying periods of abundance. In between, there are still intermittent periods of scarcity wherein *fasting*, just like millions of years ago, were considered a normal part of day to day lives. As our ancestors, they too are physically fit, active and muscular. No evidence showing signs of obesity or problems associated therewith. Causes of death are mostly related to old age, trauma in nature, accidents or infection.

This timeline comprised more than 99% of human evolution that eventually shaped our genetic make-up. The genetic changes that were incorporated during those times practically explain why our body responds instinctively the way it does, and expectedly adapted to *fasting* as it already became a normal part of life.

By the 18th century, approximately just about 200 years ago, (which is approximately a *minute part* in the overall human evolution), *advanced farming* began and a widespread availability of wheat, maize, potatoes, and rice as house staples became a norm.

With various food preservation techniques, people can now basically eat at any time they want. Food is available 24 hours a day, seven days a week, all year round. And what has become of our body that was used to scarcity and not of abundance? Did it evolve fast enough to adapt to these changes in our lifestyle brought about by industrialization? Can the human body accommodate all the modern-day food innovations that aim to prevent us all from ever experiencing hunger? Unfortunately, it did not.

Our body was stuck in an era designed for fasting. Our culinary expertise and kitchen expanded too fast for our genes to adapt. Thus, what do you think will happen to all the modern-day food that our anciently wired body is bound to consume? It actually doesn't know what to do with all that, but, store it the only way it knows how- as lots and lots of body fats. Our body kept on storing fats (just like it used to *in preparation for the inevitable days of scarcity* that was the norm for thousands of years). It stores foods in the form of fats every chance it gets in time for the supposedly *regularly occurring* or cyclic *need* for *fasting*, that, as we know now, will most likely never happen.

This food abundance is now a plague causing illnesses in various forms that usually starts with one beginning to lean towards the "healthier" side, then becomes a little overweight and before you know it, nothing fits anymore. And suddenly, you are already obese class II. From then, it can spiral down to co-morbidities associated with obesity like diabetes, hypertension, chronic back pain, arthritis, asthma, heart attack, kidney failure, stroke and many more.

You see, modern-day humans are born and raised with a mindset of avoiding hunger at all cost, by parents who were also born and raised by those who define a minimum daily activity with being able to eat at least 3 times a day. To eat even if you are not hungry simply because it is already time to eat. And what is the result? Millions are now suffering from lifestyle diseases brought about by too much and too frequent eating habits that is far from how our body is used to operate.

If only we can go back to the way we were, maybe we can have the best of the current world, with enough safety net for accidents, antibiotics for dreaded infections and a physique that can withstand all the diseases brought about by improper food intake. It may sound counterintuitive, but in an era where everyone is maximizing the availability of food, we must also do a conscious effort to limit our intake especially when we still have stored fats to lose. And by finishing this book, I hope that in a way or two, we can make it come true. ☺

CHAPTER I
Truths About Eating and Fasting

What we need to accept as humans

"Health and healing will follow fasting."

-Jentezen Franklin

Yes, the basic foundation of the *evolutionary perspective's view* in attaining our ideal weight is by incorporating fasting in our way of life.

For other people who have what we call the "skinny genes", the ones who frequents the buffet table but doesn't seem to ever gain a pound, getting fat is a far out problem, thus *fasting* simply for weight loss is not for them. This is because they belong to the

50% of the population whose genes mutated and adapted to the modern day food intake. But for many of us who have trouble attaining and maintaining a normal weight, we must accept that fasting is a natural phenomenon throughout the human existence that we must also embark on.

Living in this modern world where food comes in abundance, fasting is a taboo. Many people just cannot comprehend how one would ever consider engaging in it. People have different and often negative views and beliefs about eating and fasting that, when you investigate further, have very little scientific explanation as back up.

The following are the uncommon truths about fasting and common attitude towards food that a lot of us can benefit from knowing

- *Fasting will not kill you, eating all the time will*

If you think about it, metabolic diseases such as diabetes, heart disease, stroke and to some extent, cancers, which are all related to lifestyle and eating, cause more death than any other disease globally as published in the latest data by World Health Organization (WHO).

Although *fasting* is *not* synonymous to *starvation*, note that even the latter does't even score among the significant causes of death. If one eats 3x a day, 365 days a year, that is already 1,095 meals a year. Say you fast for a day, thus making it 1,092, do you really think it will make such negative difference in your health?

It is actually quite amusing that those who haven't fasted are those who are certain that it cannot be done. Not because they have tried it, but simply because they are not open to it.

If you come to think of it, fasting is actually being practiced by millions worldwide. It is even a part of some religious, health and philosophical disciplines. Fasting is even advocated as part of natural healing during the times of *Hippocrates*. If fasting kills, do you think humanity would survive this long?

- *Fasting will not lead to muscle wasting*

Contrary to the common misconception, fasting will not lead to muscle wasting. During our days as cavemen, our muscles are essential in our quest for food. Thus, our body adapted greatly in such a way that our muscles will not be compromised during the time that we are still looking for food and need it the most. Instead, our body has other energy sources stored specifically reserved for times like fasting. Thus, you can be sure your muscles will be well preserved.

- *Breakfast is not the most important meal of the day*

You might have heard and believed the opposite of this statement, but I hope you know that line was made popular by a company selling cereals made specifically to make breakfast convenient, with the goal of profit and not your health.

Breakfast as we know now is the meal we eat in the morning usually before 10 o'clock. And it is ok to eat it. But it is important for you to recognize why you are eating it. Is it because you haven't eaten the night before? Or you have no other time to eat the rest of the day? Or that you will engage in a very energy-requiring task that your current stores of fats cannot take? Or is it because you are just used to eating breakfast without really thinking about why?

At this point, I want you to see that eating simply because it is time to eat is not ideal and is very risky for your health. And the most important meal could be any meal, as long as you eat it when your body (*and soul*) really needs it the most.

- *Eating small frequent meals will not lead to fat loss*

When eating, it is not just the actual calories that make you gain weight. Whenever you eat, your pancreas secretes ***insulin*** and turns **on** the **fat-storing mechanism switch** in your body. Thus, eating small frequent meals will not lead to weight loss simply because you will have persistent high insulin level in your blood, making you in a state of ***perpetual fat-storing mode*** and <u>never in a fat-losing state</u>.

Any amount of weight loss some experiences are due to water loss and are usually just temporary.

- *Eating low fat, low calorie diet lowers metabolism*

Metabolism is unique for each individual. It is a function of both body composition and activity. Unfortunately, eating a low calorie, low fat diet for a long time won't boost your metabolism, instead will only make it slower. Prolonged intake of such low calorie diet will have detrimental effect both on your metabolism and overall well-being as what happened in the subjects in a starvation experiment done among males who were fed on low calorie, and mostly carbohydrate diet. (*see appendix A*)

- *The symptoms of "hypoglycemia" when skipping meals are caused by other factors other than low blood sugar*

One of the common fears of people on fasting is the risk of having a hypoglycemic episode or critically low level of blood sugar. While a low blood sugar is good especially once you are already adapted to fasting and are relying on a fuel source other than sugar *(yes, you can still live normally even if your sugar is low because it is not the only kind of fuel your body can use to function)*, the commonly feared symptoms consisting of dizziness, tremors and weakness are not actually due to hypoglycemia. These are mainly due to dehydration and/or electrolyte imbalance. *Fasting* for less than 24 hours rarely cause worrisome result. When doing an extended fast, electrolytes-rich supplements are recommended for those who will continue to engage in normal physical daily activity. Doing so will make fasting adaptation a breeze. Specifics will be discussed in the succeeding chapters.

- *Fasting doesn't make you malnourished, over-eating will*

Malnourishment refers to both being underweight and overweight. As fasting leads to weight loss, there is little evidence that it can lead to undernourishment simply because it is a voluntary process. Thus, when one already attains their goal weight, they can simply break their fast; establish a normal eating habit in such a way that they maintain their ideal weight. On the other hand, over eating as evidenced by steadily increasing number of lifestyle diseases, simply signifies improper and unhealthy kind of nourishment.

- *Fasting is healthy when done right*

Weight loss may be the most noticeable effect of fasting, but it is not the only benefit you can get. Research shows that fasting can lead to longevity, can reverse diabetes and hypertension, decrease tumor growth, heal diseases related to inflammation and even lessen the risk of developing cancer, among many others. For you to know the details on how to fast safely and effectively is the goal of this book.

CHAPTER 2
Fat-Storing Versus Fat-Losing Mechanism

Understanding how fats are made and burned

"The best of all medicines are resting and fasting."

-Benjamin Franklin

As plain as it may sound, consuming more than what your body needs will lead to weight gain in the form of fats. Each person has his own **Basal Metabolic Rate** (BMR), also known as required resting energy expenditure. This is the amount of calories your body is burning even if you are not doing anything. These calories will be needed by your thinking brain, pumping heart, working liver, digesting intestines, breathing lungs, warmth in your skin and all the other parts of your body, even while you are sleeping. At an average, BMR is about 25kcal/kg of body weight. Your BMR will dictate the minimum caloric requirement you need even when you are doing nothing. Any additional physical or mental work or any form of stress will need additional energy thereby increasing your caloric requirement.

Say for example a 35 years old woman within normal BMI, weighing 55kg and stands 5'5" with a very sedentary lifestyle will have a BMR of 1,555 kcal. If she continuous to consume more than her daily BMR, those excess foods will pile up and become body fats.

Since it is not a common practice to calculate food intake on a day to day basis, more often than not, we eat more than the amount we need. Unknowingly, the lady in our example can slide from normal to overweight line without noticing when it actually happened.

If you were able to perfectly balance your food intake, BMR and physical activity since you were young, and do not have any metabolic problems, most likely you are at your most ideal body weight and are no longer in need of this book for weight-management purposes.

However, if you are like me who have been piling up fats in all places in the course of living this beautiful life, you will realize that even if you try to eat less, the fats just don't go away. There may be times you feel that after a few days of "*dieting*" you lose weight, but the moment you go back to your normal eating habits, all the weight just comes back in. Thus, as a result, you stop what you do, continue to eat and be frustrated with how your body is transforming. It is because the initial weight loss is not true fat loss but just water loss. Because you see, the moment that you have stored fats, those fats become the least accessible form of energy that cannot be easily burned with simple reduction in food intake.

It is during this time that you must consider reducing not the amount of food that you eat, but more importantly, reducing the frequency of your meals. We have to understand that no matter how much we are used to eating all the time, it is simply NOT how nature intends our body to function, thus the weight gain we hate so badly becomes inevitable.

In addition, we have to understand that as impossible as it may seem, the less calorie you eat does not mean the more fats you will lose. The concept of *calorie in, calorie out* does not apply in the long run. Our body functions way more complex than this mechanism. Converting foods that we eat and fats in our hips into energy doesn't happen in an instant, but, ample time is necessary for this to occur. This can be understood by looking at a very simple but very important diagram below. Wherein, contrary to the common knowledge, sugar, in the form of glucose or carbohydrates is not the only source of energy for us to function efficiently. And skipping meals, even for days, will not lead to death. If you are here to lose the excess fats fast, then you have to accept that you need to do more than just reducing your carbohydrate intake. Simply put, we have to go back on how our ancestors lived their lives before. With science to back it up, we have to be accepting of the fact that fasting is an integral part of the human's way of life throughout evolution. This can be further understood by knowing the types of *fuel expenditure* our body use during different *periods of fasting*. In simpler words, this only means that your energy source will change as days go by without eating. The energy currency in your body is *Adenosine triphosphate (ATP) molecule*. And it will come from a different energy source depending on where you are at a given point in time. And yes, glucose is not your only source of energy.

DAY 1: First day without food intake, your body will scrape off all the carbohydrates you have left in your blood stream, known as your blood glucose, and the remaining ones in your stomach and intestines from your last meal. The energy from glucose is obtained through a process called **glycolysis**.

This will be enough to fuel your daily activity. Note that you will feel hungry, but not the entire day. Instead, you will only feel hungry for about 3-4 times a day depending on how you frequently take your usual meals. The hunger you will experience are proof of how wired you are to eating at least three meals a day. If you do not give in to the growling sounds of your stomach, it will subside after about an hour. You should not worry on hyperacidity since food is the primary trigger for acid secretions. If you avoid food, including seeing and smelling food, secretions of gastric acids will be suppressed. Your fuel source as of this time is carbohydrates/glucose, the red line in the graph. Drink water whenever you feel hungry, since thirst has the same symptoms as hunger. Each cycle of glycolysis will yield 2 ATP for energy.

DAY 2: At approximately 24-48 hours of fasting, your blood glucose is already depleted. This time, it will tap your glucose stores in the form of glycogen mainly found in your liver. This glycogen will be broken down into glucose through the process of **glycogenolysis**, and the glucose will again undergo glycolysis as it did on the first day. Thus, your fuel source is still carbohydrates. And depending on the amount of your glycogen stores (about 2,000 kcal on average), or your physical activity, the rate of depletion follows as you see in the decline in the red line in the graph. You will still feel hungry, but again, only during your usual eating times. Some feel they are hungrier on this day than the previous day, while others feel that the hunger sensation is starting to lessen. Once you are able to overcome the first 48 hours, chances are, the subsequent days will be easier.

DAY 3: Within 48-72 hours of fasting, you will no longer have glucose in your system, the fuel source that your body has been used to consuming for the longest time. As of this point, it will tap the next easiest source of energy in your body and create its own glucose and the substrates or *ingredients* will come from fats (the glycerol from triglycerides) and amino acids which will come from your muscles. I know you might not feel comfortable that the probably little muscles you have will be compromised. Note that it is only very minimal and will not last for long simply because your body, brilliant as it is, knows that it is not sustainable. This process called **gluconeogenesis** or the making of new glucose from your own free triglycerides/fats and muscle stores, is only an emergency fund, and not designed for long-term use because it will eventually make you weak (temporarily). In fact, some may feel weak at this point and may already want to give up.

But it is during this time that you have to hang on and take some electrolytes so your weakness, perceived or otherwise, will be relieved. As they say, rest or even sleep if you must, but do not quit. Gluconeogenesis will require 4 ATPs to occur, in order to obtain glucose for glycolysis that will only yield 2 ATPs. At this point, you can see that this process is not sustainable simply because the net ATP is negative and our body is not wired to self-destruct.

DAY 4 and up: About 72-96 hours of fasting, your body already senses that no food is going to arrive anytime soon. Thus, it will tap its stored energy from your precious vault of fats. Yes, finally, it will use up your fats as its primary energy source. This process is called **lypolysis**, which simply means, breakdown of lipids.

As of this point, the real and major fat breakdown occurs.

Fat's usable energy form is called ketone bodies (indicated by the green line in the graph). This is also known as **Ketosis** or the shifting of energy stores from glucose to ketones. Ketone bodies are very energy-dense molecules wherein one ketone body will yield 22 ATPs. This explains why there are so many testimonials saying that after days of fasting, they felt a sense of increased strength and energy and even improved mental prowess. **Ketones** are actually the preferred fuel source by many organs, including the brain, and once adapted in *Ketosis,* even the other organs like muscles can now utilize ketones as an efficient energy source. For some, there is this stage of *Ketoflu*, wherein one experiences signs and symptoms of flu without having actual flu because the body is still adjusting. This is because our body is not used to using ketones as a fuel, and simply because, just like every other regular human, we've never really and truly *fast* our entire lives. But on days 4-5, hunger is already at minimum though you can still feel it occurring the same time on the previous days, but this time, it won't bother you anymore because the hunger hormone *Ghrelin* is already declining.

Note that there may be an overlap among these biochemical processes. Some studies indicate that ketosis starts to occur as early as 12 hours of fasting with heavy ketosis occurring at 18 hours.

For some people and even other fellow doctors, the mere mention of ketosis already signifies a big red flag. This is because basic biochemistry books in medical school discuss ketosis very briefly and it is always subsequently alongside starvation and diabetic *ketoacidosis,* which can be fatal.

However, they failed to emphasize that the ketoacidosis occurs when there is a persistently high level of blood glucose together with high level of ketones among diabetic patients whose food intake is largely composed of sugar and/or absence of insulin to regulate the sugar within the blood stream. However, for those who are non-diabetics, fasting will follow the normal transition of fuel source (carbohydrate to fats), thus blood glucose will decrease and only ketones will increase to a nutritional level where weight loss is achieved. Blood ketone level for steady weight loss is at approximately 1.0-3.0mmol/L when doing short extended fasts. Whereas heavy ketosis and greater weight loss effects are achieved during prolonged extended fast and even this seldom reach more than 5.0mmol/L. Even at more elevated levels, it will NOT cause acidosis because ketones are naturally produced when fat burning mechanism ensues. The dangerous level of ketoacidosis is at 10mmol/L and occurs together with elevated blood glucose as a complication of type 1 diabetes.

As of this point, your blood sugar and insulin are at a stable level and in the lower range of normal, where they should always be.

According to *Loren Lockman*, advocate of water fasting and one who supervised thousands of long-term extended fasts, an average person has the capacity to do a safe water-only fasting for up to six weeks. That as long as you have fat stores and your body fat percentage does not go down below 5-12%, you can live with energy coming from ketones & gluconeogenesis only. The longest recorded fast in a medical journal is 382 days and the subject stopped when he finally reached his ideal weight. He sustained the weight loss and had normal BMI throughout his life.

I know at this point you might have doubts, especially with your capacity to do it. I know because I myself had doubts too, because in my 30 years of existence I have never had a day where I had not had any food.

But after thorough research and scientific boosting of confidence, I trusted the process. I decided to put my faith in nature, knowing that fasting has been an integral part of human evolution and it is a practice of almost all religions from time immemorial. I started my first 5 days of water-only fasting relying not on how I was raised, or what the media advertisements says, but on the evolutionary perspective's scientific confidence why fasting can be done safely and smoothly. I trusted the fact that because our genes have been through thousands of years of experience, it enabled our body to sustain it.

Surprisingly, not known to many, our body is more adapted to scarcity than gluttony. And as I went through the fasting days, with psychological turmoil going on inside my head, I found solace knowing that regular extended fasting has been a way of life of millions of people all over the world. Miles and miles away from where I live, people are connecting and supporting each other during extended fasting. Hundreds of blogs and videos discuss the benefits of fasting and even documenting their daily update during an active fast.

I successfully completed a 5-day water-only fast while continuously and properly working in the hospital doing my usual ward/ER routine and surgeries. From the food glutton that I was, I became liberated from food dependency. From seeking food all the time, my mental strength has never been better. I felt like a totally different person, that I have achieved a certain level of elation that nothing else can give. It is a level of confidence and empowerment that only you can give yourself. If I can do it, I know you can too. Imagine a few days of psychological exercise in exchange of finally attaining the body you've always been dreaming of.

Fasting can be done in various schedules and lengths. With proper guidance from this book, anybody can do it at his or her own convenience and keep on doing it until they reach their ideal body image. And you do not need to do the whole four days or more, not even a full 24 hours because there are smoother ways to reach ketosis other than engaging in a prolonged fast.

Want it and it will be yours. Trust that it can be done. Write down how much you want it and why you want to have that ideal body. Focus on that goal and let it be your fuel to give *fasting* a try. There is nothing else better than you being in control of both your body and your mind.

SUMMARY of STAGES of FASTING

Day 1: Fuel source is from Blood Sugar/Glucose, hunger pangs is severe; this can lead to lowering of your blood sugar and water loss as well.

Day 2: Fuel Source is from Sugar/Glucose coming from the storage form Glycogen mostly from the liver, hunger may decrease but may be worse for some; this will deplete the glycogen in the liver

Day 3: Fuel source is mostly from glucose made from breakdown of fats (triglycerides) and muscles, some ketones are produced from breakdown of fats, this can lead to fat loss and minimal muscle loss

Day 4 and beyond: Major fuel source is now ketones, which came from your fat stores, hunger at its lowest and this is the stage where pure fat loss occurs and blood sugar and insulin is low but stable.

CHAPTER 3

Why Meal Timing Matters

Recognizing "when to eat" is the key

"If anything is worth doing, do it with all your heart."

-Buddha

Fasting is essential to strike a balance in one's way of life. However, it is not sustainable for you to keep on fasting all throughout, because then, no balance shall result. This is the point where we answer the question: when should we really eat in order for us to get back the eating equilibrium our generation has lost?

And the answer is "No, it's not your usual breakfast-lunch-dinner routine. Nor is it is the kindergarten's *breakfast - morning snacks - lunch -*

afternoon snacks - dinner - bedtime milk time". When to eat, should actually be something instinctive. Like the animals in the wild, we humans are supposed to eat only when we are hungry and stop eating when we are full. Following these instincts, no-one should become overweight (except for special natural occurrences like pregnancy and growth of a child). So, if this is the case, when did we go wrong? Why is obesity starting to become a worldwide pandemic, especially among the resource-sufficient parts of the world?

Unfortunately, this comes down with nature versus nurture. For our generation, unfortunately, nurture took reign. Remember when you were forced to eat as a child even when you don't want to? Or when you were forced to stay in the dinner table until you finish everything your mother put on your plate? No, it's not your parent's fault. Because like almost everyone in this planet plagued by the marketing strategies of the multi-billion food industry, parents too are fooled by statements like, "Breakfast is the most important meal of the day" or "Always be ready, never go hungry" schemes.

As it turned out, those hard-to-put-on-breakfast-table kids are actually the ones we should follow. Those kids are listening and responding to their instincts, that they should eat only when their bodies are already in need of nutrition and they stop when they've had enough. However, with constant *reward-punishment parenting model* we adults unknowingly give, plus the undeniable pleasure from sweets and simple sugars, those instincts are eventually lost. By nature, hunger hormone *Ghrelin* increases when your body is truly hungry (as in lacking energy and resources to finish a certain task). However, over time, *Ghrelin* increases simply because the body is used to receiving food during specific times of the day despite the abundant food storage in our bodies in the form of fats.

Studies show that during a 24-hour monitoring, *Ghrelin* increases in response to the usual eating routine and corresponds to the hunger pangs a person is experiencing when not giving in to the hunger sensation occasioned by this hormone.

And it is important to note that overtime, contrary to the common knowledge, one does not get hungrier as the time passes. Instead, the sense of hunger will pass after about an hour and will only recur during the next meal time, with just about the same or even lesser hunger sensation than before, as seen in the graph below indicating a declining *Ghrelin* level as the days of fasting go by. If one eats, especially when eating low carbohydrate diet with minimal protein and high in healthy fats, the fullness hormone *Leptin* increases and this signals your brain to stop eating. This is the reason why animals in the wild don't become obese, because there is a balance between *Ghrelin* and *Leptin* in their body and they respond to it accordingly.

So, how can we re-establish a balanced and well-functioning *Ghrelin* and *Leptin*? Simple, just unlearn what you have learned. That is, intentionally disrupting the eating pattern you've been used to your whole life. By not responding to the urge to eat just because it's 12 noon, and to consciously refuse food intake when you know you still have a lot of fats in store. Yes, in a word, what you need to do is *fast*. In order to regain your instinctive drive, you can slowly reset your body to its natural state. Fasting is the key to **appetite correction** or the reestablishment of balance between *Leptin and Ghrelin hormones*. There's a rapid way, and there's a smooth slow way. But if significant weight loss is your goal, then, you can go for the highway - in this case, scheduled fasting.

CHAPTER 4
The Basics of Fasting

Must-knows every future faster needs

"The secret of change is to focus all of your energy, not on fighting the old, but on building the new."

-Socrates

To embark on the highway option, the first thing you need to do is to know what fasting really means. As described in the founder of Intensive Dietary Management and Nephrologist, *Dr. Jason Fung*, in his books: *The Obesity Code* and (co-author *Jim Moore*) *the Complete Guide to Fasting*, it is clearly explained that fasting is not synonymous to starvation. **Fasting** is the voluntary non-consumption or omission of calorie-containing food and beverages. Whereas, **starvation,** is the involuntary absence or negation of food intake, despite the person's protest or natural need for food sustenance. Although they may initially affect one's physical aspects similarly, the large difference is on the emotional and psychological impact each has. With starvation, detrimental effects of feeling of vulnerability and helplessness can ensue. Whereas in fasting, the person is in control, he is totally in charge, empowering him for every hour endured knowing that one can break it anytime as desired. Fasting has impacted those who practice it not just physically, but also mentally and spiritually and in a good way.

There are so many fasting schedules available for everyone (*daily basis or weekly*) and you can study them and see which fasting routine can work for you.

As hard to believe as it may seem, the struggle in fasting is actually 95% psychological and only 5% physical.

In general, fasting is considered **fasting** if you have not taken any calorie containing food and drinks for at least 12 hours. Studies show that after 12 hours, ketosis or breakdown of fats already start. And by the 18th hour, you are already in heavy ketosis where a large part of your energy is coming from ketones. If you extend it to 24 hours, other health-enhancing benefits occur, but the most important of which, as of this point, is the commencement of the burning of heavily-guarded and highly stubborn stored fats. The longer you fast, the more stubborn fats you lose. It's that simple.

During your fasting period, you can consume as much water, natural tea or black coffee you want, especially if you fast less than 24 hours. This is called a *Clean Fast* and is something that I advocate whenever I engage in a daily intermittent fast or short-term extended fast. You should always be mindful with how your body responds and you should keep yourself hydrated.

However, prolonged fasting can sometimes lead to electrolyte-imbalance in certain people, especially that a significant amount of electrolytes are continuously eliminated in urine. Thus, in order to avoid such occurrence, consumption of electrolyte and micronutrient-containing liquids are allowed as long as it does not contain any calorie nor it has a sweet taste like artificial sweeteners. Only zero-calorie liquids that contain electrolytes may be consumed, especially during prolonged fasting. Examples include water, coffee, tea, vinegar with or without salt and electrolytes.

As identified by Gin Stephen's book *"Delay, Don't Deny"*, any additional consumption is already classified as *dirty fasting* and such is not advisable because even if you do not eat any solid foods, consumption of any calorie-containing liquid or even zero-calorie foodstuff having a sweet taste can already stop the fat-burning processes seen in *Clean Fasting*.

However, according to *Dr. Jason Fung*, during an *extended fast of more than 24 hours* ,certain amount of good fats may be incorporated in addition to the previously stated allowed fluids, whenever one feel really weak but doesn't want to break the fast. These include coconut oil, heavy whipped cream, medium-chain triglyceride oil, or bone and vegetable broth. These additions will not jeopardize your fasting state because these fat-rich substance will still chemically mimic fasting, thus, will not kick one out of ketosis.

Personally, I recommend doing a clean water-only fasting for as long as you can. If there comes a point of feeling weak, one can consume salt water and magnesium supplements since those are the electrolytes that are frequently lost. If the weakness persists and continue to worsen, dirty fasting may be done by consuming any pure natural fats or bone broth. Note that consuming anything with flavor, even if it has zero calories, can trigger hunger more, thus you have to be careful with what you choose to consume during your fasting. Details on the fluids you can take during fasting will be discussed the next chapter.

As previously discussed, each stage of fasting will have a different effect on one's body. This is the best time to review the summary of stages of fasting and the corresponding fuel source being utilized as first seen in Chapter 2.

CHAPTER 5

Fluids You Can Take While Fasting

Water is the best of all

"The noblest of all studies is the study of what man is and of what life he should live."

-Plato

During fasting, fluids are your best friends. One can survive months of no food intake, but three days without water can already cause serious problems.

Of all fluids there is, the most important of all is luckily the cheapest, which is, water. Distilled water is the purest, but any unflavored water may also do.

Water-only fast has proven to be the best if your central aim is pure fat loss because intake of anything that needs metabolizing will take up energy from your body. With water-only fast, you are practicing your body to function at its optimum and in the most efficient way. Without any flavor that passes through your gut, you are able to provide rest to your bowels, pancreas and the rest of your gastrointestinal tract. Upon introduction to your system, water will enable the very basic processes of converting glucose, glycogen and fats into energy that may be used for daily tasks and for facilitating fat loss.

During fasting it is very important that you take time to listen to your body. Identify temporary hunger pangs due to routine eating time versus hunger due to true nutrient deficiency.

Always have water in hand as it is important to be kept hydrated. However, it is also equally important not to "over hydrate" by consuming water way more than what you need. Over hydration may be suspected if you experience frequent urination, and is experienced almost immediately after water intake with the same or more amount than you took, followed by episodes of worsening muscle weakness. This is because water and sodium go together as they are eliminated in your urine. And as your body is still not used to fasting, it has the tendency to eliminate them both, not knowing that the kidneys must save all the electrolytes it can gather. As a result, you will become sodium-deficient or *hyponatremic* which will manifest as weakness, easy fatigability and light-headedness. But, if you listen to your body carefully, and by drinking sips of water, little by little only, whenever you feel thirsty or hungry, and avoid gulping liters in one setting, can eliminate the risk of *over-hydration* complications.

However, if such symptoms still occur, it is at this point that you can add non-caloric substance to your water that cannot break your fast and will not aggravate hunger but can help you sustain your fasting commitment. These are essential electrolytes that get deficient during prolonged fasting with normal day to day activity. In my case, I find that a teaspoon of vinegar, mixed with a pinch of salt & diluted with two tablespoons of water, suppresses my appetite and gives me an energy boost from sodium replacement.

(Some water-only fasting advocates are not promoting the incorporation

of supplement but are advising total bed rest during this period.)

When fasting for 1-2 weeks, sodium, magnesium, and to some extent, potassium supplements, will suffice. However, for longer fasts, additional supplementation of calcium, chloride and phosphorous is necessary to avoid risk of *re-feeding syndrome*.

Below is a list of common electrolytes important in fasting and corresponding symptoms of deficiency.

1.   Salt

Sodium as the basic chemical component of salt is the most

abundant electrolyte in our body. It is one of the most common components for humans to perform regular functions, and its most important organ regulator of which is our kidneys. When one has more sodium, kidneys just simply eliminate it through urine and when the same is depleting, the kidney will try to keep whatever amount it can save before urinating. However, it is not that easy to perfect the optimum water intake, and to teach kidneys to readily save all the salts you have during your first few days of fasting. Thus, to slowly introduce the transition, you can prepare and infuse your body with home-made salt water, and taking sips when necessary. (*Again, I find that mixing salt, water and vinegar is more palatable than salt and water alone.)* You will be amazed that you can immediately feel some improvement on your strength after you take a sip. The more organic the salt, the better it is. Good reviews were handed to pink Himalayan salts, but I find any pure, organic sea salt to perform the job just as fine. To make your own concoction, just take 1 tablespoon of salt and mix it with 50-500 ml of water. Whatever amount left that day should be discarded and make another one for the next day. Or, simply have a pinch of salt to your tongue and flush it with water as needed. Signs and symptoms of low sodium or *hyponatremia* include muscle cramps, loss of appetite and dizziness. These symptoms are often attributed to *hypoglycemia* or low blood sugar, but more often than not, it is just due to low salt in the body. Thus, if this happens, take some and see the improvements after.

2. Magnesium

While magnesium is commonly disregarded, it is in fact very important in processes that involve electrical impulses in the body, particularly in the muscles, nerves and heart. Symptoms of deficiency will include muscular cramps and spasms, difficulty to concentrate and palpitations. During the first 1-3 days, seldom does hypomagnesemia occur.

But as your fasting progresses and you start to feel these symptoms to occur, you can consider taking in magnesium supplements at 200 to 400 mg per day. Personally, I only noticed symptoms of muscle cramps on the 10th day of water only fasting. This may vary from person to person depending on you bodily stores.

3.   Potassium

This is the second most important ion in the body. It functions hand in hand with sodium. And since sodium loss is expected especially during the early phase of fasting, potassium loss or *hypokalemia* can also ensue.

Symptoms of hypokalemia can include muscle weakness, blood pressure changes and mental confusion. Thus, it is optimum to have potassium supplements in handy when engaging in extended fast (>5-7 days). The amount you need will depend on your physical activity. If you are an athlete or doing heavy physical labor, you can consider taking in a little more than the recommended daily allowance of 1,500-2,000 mg for the average adult. However, for those that are not engaging in strenuous activities, potassium is seldom required even in extended fasts of more than 5-7 days.

Aside from those, there are also other electrolytes that are needed in small amount but seldom causes problems unless you are very physically active or doing resistance training or already has signs of osteoporosis. These include calcium, chloride (already part of salt as sodium chloride), bicarbonate, phosphorous and phosphates. However, if you are still young without co-morbidities and are not engaging in laborious routine, you can proceed without taking much of the latter supplements. On the other hand, if you feel you need them, further readings are suggested.

Remember, electrolyte deficiency is the most common cause of *Ketoflu*, and a resultant termination of fasting. It is of great importance to prepare and properly equip yourself prior to embarking on an extended fast in order for you to be fully prepared and attain success in this journey.

Other than electrolytes, other non-caloric additions can improve the fasting experience. This is considered a clean fast.

1. Coffee - whether with or without caffeine, as long as there is no sugar or cream is a good addition to your water. It boosts your metabolism and a great option for those who are avid coffee drinkers. For those who are not used to taking in black

coffee (i.e. no sugar or cream), you can start taking it as light as possible and slowly increase the strength to suit your taste.

2. Tea - any organic tea leaves is okay to add flavor to your water in addition to the inherent properties of individual teas (i.e. green tea's appetite suppression, calming effect of chamomile, caffeine-fix of black teas).

3. Zero calorie spices like cinnamon, ginger or turmeric are also welcome, however, carefully consider prior to adding these since flavor instantly triggers appetite and

subsequent hunger sensation might result.

Water with electrolytes is the best fluid you can take in achieving functional, energy-sufficient fasting days. Fasting without any fluids, which is called dry fasting is strongly DISCOURAGED.

When engaging in your first extended fast, I suggest keeping it as clean as possible, as whatever length of time you clock in, is already a lifetime worth of personal achievement that you can take pride and make reference to. For instance, a week-long water-only fasting, is a bragging record and a motivational reference for your future self that if you can do it that one time, surely you can do it again and can readily take on any other less challenging tasks, and mind you, there are too many less challenging tasks than saying no to any amount and any type of food for days.

On the other hand, below are the fluids you can consume while on dirty fasting mode as advised by Dr. Jason Fung in his book entitled, *The Obesity Code and The Complete Guide to Fasting*. These fluids have high fat and nutrient contents, that even if you are truly already breaking your fast, "biochemically" you are still fasting because you would be utilizing fats/ketones still, thus, you are not getting out of ketosis stage or the fat burning stage and you can proceed with your body fat loss thereafter.

1. Vegetable Broth - the soup from cooked vegetables and spices. Strain the vegetables and drink the soup only. It contains electrolytes and some salt to quench your thirst and to some extent, hunger. *(Dirty Fast)*

2. Bone Broth - the soup from boiled meat, preferably with bones. Strain and drink the soup especially when feeling weak during extended fasting. *(Dirty Fast)*

3. Bulletproof coffee - one cup of black coffee and froth with 1 tablespoon of fats like coconut oil, medium chain triglyceride (MCT) oil, whole milk, butter, heavy whipping cream or cinnamon for flavor. Limit to only 1-2 cups per day. *(Dirty Fast)*

4. Water with natural vinegar (apple cider or pure coconut vinegar) - shown to have good effects on appetite suppression and abdominal pain from stomach acid secretions. Mix 1 tablespoon of vinegar, with or without salt in water. Dilute as tolerated. *(Clean Fast)*

5. Water with lemons and lime or fruit slices without consuming the fruits. The citrus extracts will add flavor to water but this may contain some sugar. *(Dirty Fast)*

To recap, water with electrolytes is considered clean fasting. Other zero-calorie and non-sweet fluids like black coffee, tea and vinegar can be taken in a clean fast. Personally, I take pleasure in pure, organic zero calorie vinegar (coconut or apple cider) mixed with salt and water, which is a very good source of electrolytes and an effective appetite suppressant when fasting. Others even put some salts in their coffee, so, you can also personalize your own.

Clean fasting should be advocated for daily intermittent fast (IF) and as long as you can during extended fast (EF). Other fluid additions should only be considered when doing the latter. Differentiation between IF and EF will be discussed in the succeeding chapters.

Again, I am putting emphasis on the three types of fasting in descending order in a matter of purity and priority when fasting. First is the *water-only fasting (plus salt)*, the cleanest form of fasting and is something I believe in doing for as long as I can. Once I already feel weak or with signs of electrolyte imbalance, I will proceed with a *clean fasting*, wherein black coffee, tea and other electrolytes like salt can be added. Lastly, when engaging in a fast of more than 3 days, I allow myself to have *dirty fasting* when I can no longer stick to clean fasting and if I cannot sustain it, I then decide to break the fast.

CHAPTER 6
Who Can Fast

"Our souls need fasting as much as our bodies need food."

-Islamic Proverb

As we are all descendants of humanity, anybody can actually fast. In fact, everybody has fasted many times in the past without knowing it. The daily gap between your dinner and breakfast the following day is already fasting, thus the term "breakfast", or breaking a fast.

However, benefits are seen when fasting is extended to a minimum of 12 hours, just enough to rid your blood stream of all the sugars you've had the previous day. Weight loss through ketosis, starts to significantly kick in after the 16th hour and can be slowly extended to as long as tolerated.

Any adult who wants to lose weight with the right mental understanding of the risks and benefits of fasting can engage in such. Anybody who are physically able without any known illness, not taking any medications and are desirous of improving their overall health, are the best people to start this journey.

If you have illnesses and/or symptoms related to any lifestyle diseases such as obesity, chronic pain, diabetes, hypertension and elevated cholesterol, you can still engage in fasting provided you have proper guidance from your trusted physician.

The latter subgroup can actually benefit the most from fasting and studies show that these lifestyle diseases even have the potential to be reversed. Although there are a lot of success stories from those who did it on their own, it is highly advised that thorough consideration, research and preparation should be done first before engaging in any type of extended fasting.

Although in general, intermittent fasting can be smoothly done by those with maintenance medications and in need of frequent monitoring, any form of extended fast must be done with guidance or under the direct supervision of healthcare professionals since individual medical history and response vary from person to person.

However, for those with no known serious illness and without symptoms suggesting such, young or otherwise, and have extra weight to manage or reduce, then it is best to start immediately while risks are minimal and benefits are at best.

CHAPTER 7
Who Cannot Fast

"I'm not telling you it's going to be easy, I'm telling you it's going to be worth it."

-Anonymous

Fasting, especially extended fasting is not recommended among limited groups of individuals belonging in this subgroup:

1. Growing children - as they are still in their developmental years, children are prohibited from engaging in intentional and extended fasts. The nutrients from food are essential in order for them to reach physical maturity. For very young

children, their peripheral fats are essential in heat regulation to avoid hypothermia, thus, fat loss at this time is strongly discouraged. They, however, can benefit from eating in moderation and meal timing that is not dictated by routine, but by their instinctive and nutritional bodily needs.

2. Pregnant and breastfeeding women (especially those exclusively breastfeeding infants less than 4-6 months old)- this is among the most established occurrence in nature where weight gain is expected and is encouraged as this relates and

ensures the proper development of the offspring. Fasting may jeopardize both the health of the baby or the mother; and when nature is forced to choose, the latter is likely to be sacrificed.

Although there are a lot of illnesses that can be benefited by fasting, an educated and informed approach should be done before deciding on anything that can possibly put one in danger. Certain medications affect metabolism in an erratic way, and there is logic to the saying "Better safe than sorry."

Other subgroups that need precaution are as follows:

- Those on prescription medications and with diagnosed diseases- those who are currently diagnosed with any medical, especially type 1 diabetes, or psychiatric conditions are warned not to engage in fasting without prior consultation with their respective physicians.

- Those with known hyperacidity or predisposed to having stomach ulcers - although there are a number of factors that contribute to ulcer formation, an active ulcer or gastritis are sometimes aggravated by fasting. Proper treatment of hyperacidity or related illness like gastroesophageal reflux disease (GERD) and knowledge on how to counter the risk during fasting should be attained first prior to considering this course.

• Those with history of fainting spells - fainting have a lot of possible causes but the common ones include hypoglycemia, orthostatic hypotension or decrease in blood pressure from sudden positional changes and heightened parasympathetic response in times of extreme stress. Appropriate investigation must be done first prior to fasting.

- Those who are undernourished or in cachexia - severe malnutrition such as *kwashiorkor* and *marasmus*, as often seen in children in areas with famine can also be seen in adults. Cachexia manifested by being severely underweight, and wasting usually from chronic illnesses and late stage diseases are contraindicated to undergo fasting.

- Those with eating disorders - those diagnosed with eating disorders, especially anorexia are advised against fasting. Certain eating disorders that can benefit from true weight loss should consider doing so only under direct supervision of a professional.

Other specific conditions not mentioned here may be contraindicated to fast. In that case, kindly consult with your trusted physician first should you have doubts whether you can fast or not.

CHAPTER 8
Extended Fasting

"Everyone can perform magic, everyone can reach his goals, if he is able to think, if he is able to wait, if he is able to fast."

-Herman Hesse

No solid food intake for more than 24 hours is already considered an extended fast (EF). There are multiple variations of fasting that are expounded on the books written by *Dr. Jason Fung* and *Gin Stephen,* but for the sake of efficient weight loss, I believe that the most natural way is through a scheduled EF of 5 days or more mimicking how our hunter and gatherer ancestors did it before.

Although extended periods of starvation was unintentional at first, the thousands of years of repeating pattern of fasting, eating and fasting again eventually became a norm and got embedded in our system. Since our genetic make-up adapted, it enabled our body to optimize its functions even during a fasted state. In fact, evidence show that fasting has become an integral part of human's natural biochemical processes wherein absence of prolonged fasts are thought to be the root cause of a number of metabolic dysfunctions that people are suffering today.

EF's immediate effect is weight loss. And it is simply due to absence of food intake that sets your body into fat burning mode, as compared to fed state in eating wherein your body is simply in the fat-storing mode.

If you've never really fasted long enough or engage in energy-spending activities enough to activate lipolysis (fat-burning), your entire life is practically a pile up of fat-storing years leading to an existence dominated by fat-staying mechanism. Both fat-burning and fat-storage phases of our bodily functions are set in motion without our active involvement and without clear notice from our end.

A 7-day EF regime is what I recommend to those who want to jumpstart the process, know their capacity and maximize weight loss within the shortest possible time. With proper mindset and some extras to help during EF, it is said that in general, a person has an average of 6 weeks fat allowance to sustain a clean fast. Some fasting gurus say that the real magic and wonder happen after the 21st day, when tumors reduce in size, mental clarity is activated at its optimum and most medical conditions are reversed. However, for the purposes of natural and time-efficient weight loss, a minimum of seven days is what I recommend as a beginner's fasting routine. On the other hand, if your schedule will not allow as of this point, a 5-day extended fast is fairly reasonable because you will have at least a day of reaching full ketosis and fat burning level that is good enough for you to be inspired to do it again.

Below is a sample table of a seven-day fasting protocol with the corresponding preparations, expectations and results. Engaging in EF more than 7 days might require additional vitamin & mineral supplements as discussed in the previous chapters

This is a simple approximation of when glycolysis, glycogenolysis, gluconeogenesis and lipolysis/ketosis occur on average. Certain people will have variation depending on their glycogen and muscle stores.

Although I highly recommend a 5-7-day jumpstart EF, you can design it to fit your own lifestyle, either longer or shorter. It is said that when your hunger starts to recur especially when there's no trigger like visual or smell stimulation, that is a good sign to break your fast, regardless of your fasting schedule.

Again, variations of dirty fasting may be opted but I personally do not recommend such especially before you know how you can really perform on a clean fast. Like this sample schedule:

Day 1 and 2: Expect to be at your hungriest, take only water and salt whenever you feel hungry, thirsty or light-headed. Rest and lie down if necessary.

Day 3-5: Hunger is more tolerable, you can add magnesium 1-2 tablets per day.

Day 6-7: Hunger may occasionally be more prominent, make sure you are well hydrated. If you have muscle pains/cramps despite adequate sodium and magnesium, you can add potassium on this day.

A question of when to do it is also as important. And for me, the answer is the soonest that you can. If you do not have important events where food intake is inevitable like a wedding in the family, birthday of someone special or a golden wedding anniversary, then fasting can be done immediately. In fact, you can do it during your most routine week and some even suggest doing it when you are expecting to be at your busiest. That way, your mind will be taken away from food and your body will easily shift on "hunting" mode thereby increasing your focus and concentration. And before you know it, your day is already done.

As I have previously mentioned, the challenge in fasting is basically 95% psychological and only 5% physical. That 95% can easily be countered by equipping yourself with the knowledge that you are truly physiologically capable. Mentally prepare yourself for all the expected manifestations of fasting and embrace episodes of hunger knowing that such negative sensation is only staying for a fleeting moment, and the 5% physical struggle can even be less. To discuss more on the types of EF and their applicability in certain situations, here are the common variations:

1. ADF or Alternate Day Fasting - this is when you fast for a day, proceed with a regular eating window hours the next day and fast the next alternatively. If you eat regularly at the same time, this will give you a 36-hour fasting and 12-hour eating window every 2 days. This can be done when one already reaches a normal BMI but wanted to lose pounds little by little to a more comfortable and lighter body without engaging in longer fasts.

2. 24 hour fasting protocol - when one engages in a 24-hour fasting every other day,

equivalent to 3 cycles per week. This protocol can be done during maintenance phase for those who are always busy. This way, time can be maximized since food preparation is reduced to once every other day.

3. 42 Hour fasting protocol - in this schedule, you have a 6-hour eating window every other day, providing a 42-hour fasting in between. This is usually done by those with very slow metabolism in order for them to jumpstart weight loss without engaging in even longer fasts. This is also perfect for those who have a very busy day to day

schedule who wants to maximize their time without getting bothered by food intake every now and then.

4. Extended fasting for more than 3 days - is usually done after a prolonged planned indulgence like holidays or vacations, or to break a plateau or to jumpstart on ketosis every now and then. For EF for weight loss, journey it with me in Appendix G. (See sample weekly schedule)

Note that during the first try, when you are not yet adapted to fasting, there will be signs of hypoglycemia that usually accompany your hunger pangs. This will include tremors, cold sweats, and some degree of light headedness. If this occurs, you can rest for a while, drink water with salt and observe. If persists, you can add magnesium or take bone broth and see if it will improve. On the other hand, if your condition is continue to worsen, immediately terminate fasting and slowly introduce food to your system. Note that for some, it may take several attempts to successfully complete a planned EF, and there is no shame in that. Each attempt will have a benefit of its own and the eventual success will be worth it.

Other unpleasant but harmless changes that may occur during EF are as follows:

1. Absent or reduced bowel movement
2. Body odor or bad "acetone" breath from ketosis
3. Headache during the early phase (~3-5 days)
4. Sleep disturbance or shortened sleep cycle

These "side effects" can easily be managed and seldom cause problems, especially that the benefits strongly outweigh those risks. However, if this is not enough to convince you to do an extended fast, then by all means, don't. Extended fasting is not the exclusive way to lose weight. But it is the fastest and most natural way to do it. And I find it very useful in keeping the fat loss I already accomplished. Note that sustaining the weight loss will need the normalization of hunger and satiety hormones, which can be achieved by breaking the lifelong frequent eating routine so many of us are used to.

Multiple *EFs* may be done before one can reach their ideal weight. However, if after trying and EF is something that you cannot do outright, do not worry because there is still a way to lose those extras long-term. For a slower yet smoother weight loss transition, intermittent fasting can be done instead.

CHAPTER 9
Intermittent Fasting

"Periodic fasting can help clear up the mind and strengthen the body and the spirit."

-Ezra Taft Benson

Simply known as IF, unknown to many, it has different variations. If this is the first time that you have heard of it and is not too sure that you can do it, you can make assessment by mentally counting the hours from the time you usually have your dinner at night, and the time you have your breakfast in the morning. If it is less than 12 hours, then you can slowly extend it to 12 by either having dinner early or moving your breakfast a little later the next day. Remember that your bedtime milk or hot cocoa counts, so you can also start by skipping that or drinking chamomile tea instead. Slowly, you can increase your fasting period by the hour each day.

Once you get the hang of it, you can proceed until you reach 16 hours fasting and an 8 hour eating window where you can eat as normally as you would. That is called a 16:8 schedule which is the most common variation. You can adjust your eating window based on your work schedule or daily routine. With a minimum of 16 hours fast and a maximum of 8 hours of eating window, you can skip at least 1 major meal, like breakfast or dinner. At first you may tend to overeat during your window, but overtime, you should learn that the time lost in fasting doesn't mean a time lost on eating that you should compensate after. Instead, think of it as a time well-spent allowing your body to burn fat, and those undesirable fats that luckily got burned, need not be replaced.

You will be surprised at how easy it is, especially when you are at your busiest in the morning, to skip breakfast and even lunch. After a month or so, you can lengthen it to 18:6 or even 20:4. It is important that you listen to your body when you eat. Don't eat simply because your window is open. Instead, eat slowly when you are hungry and stop the moment you feel satisfied. An 8-hour eating window does not mean an 8-hour of nonstop eating. Instead, you can plan 2 proper meals with or without a light snack in between.

As you move your fasting window longer, know that the benefits are also multiplying by the hour. The 19:5 is advocated by Dr. Atkin in his book where he noted that by reducing your eating window to 5 hours, you can skip two meals, making it a One Meal A Day routine or OMAD. This can also be done in 20:4 schedules. Some even do it as long as 22:2 but this has a risk of lowering your overall metabolism, thus, I personally do not recommend doing it on a daily basis. What is great about fasting is that it is very flexible especially during special occasions or dinner out where you can simply adjust on a day to day basis so long as you do not go below what I consider the minimum 16 hours regular fasting. Always count your fasting hours starting from the last food intake of the previous day.

Again, note that OMAD does not mean a single meal alone. You can open your window by having some light snacks, like a salad or a soup, an avocado or 2 poached eggs. After 30 minutes or an hour, you can proceed with your main meal with your choice of meat or whatever that you are happy with. And just before closing your window, you can drink some coffee and some nuts and cheese if you still feel like it.

OMAD is known to break the *Ghrelin-Leptin* hormonal imbalance most people are suffering in this modern day. It is also one of the best ways to maintain your fat loss once you've reached your goal weight. Other benefits include appetite correction, regularization of bowel movement, economical, more time and focus on other important matters and more freedom from food choices.

CHAPTER 10
What Can Jeopardize Fat Loss & Fasting

"The discipline of fasting breaks you out of the world's routine."

-Jentezen Franklin

If there is one word that you need to know in this weight loss journey, it should be that very word that jeopardizes fasting and fat loss, and that is, insulin. Insulin is the hormone that is released whenever you take in food. It is essential but it should be kept at a lower level since fluctuations can easily lead to weight gain. Because the moment it is circulated in your blood stream, your body sets off all the mechanisms of being in a *fed state,* and that would mean fat storage.

Insulin spike sends signal to your brain that it is the time of abundance, like the harvest season, or a successful hunting trip, in human's early evolution. Thus, our body being remarkably amazing and frugal as it is will save all the extra food you eat and store it in the form of glycogen and fats for future fasting use.

Generally, all calorie-containing foods and to some extent, zero calorie sweeteners trigger insulin secretion, but in a hierarchy, carbohydrates is the most potent stimulus, followed by proteins and the least stimuli of all, fats. Thus, consumption of any of those can break your fast and eventually jeopardize the fat loss in fasting. It is the reason why avoidance of food must be done at all cost during fasting in order for you to see the results you are trying to achieve. Note that you can eat again during your window, but fat loss is maximized if you consume healthy and fatty food (instead of carbohydrates) even during your eating window.

It is at this point that we will discuss the basic truths about the food we consume so that we can better understand and maneuver our ways both during fasting and feasting periods.

Food can be divided into three macronutrients, namely Carbohydrates, Proteins and Fats. In general:

Carbohydrates include bread, rice, pasta, potatoes, cereals, cakes, pastries and most fruits. They are known to give us energy and back in our grade school days, they were the ones that populated the **Go** part in the *go, grow and glow food chart.* Chemistry-wise, its basic unit is **Glucose**, in layman's term, this simply equates to **sugar.** Remember, excess carbohydrates are stored as glycogen and glycogen has very limited storage space largely in the liver. Consuming extra carbohydrates after your glycogen is full leads to fat stores. Physiologically speaking, there is no such thing as essential carbohydrate, simply because, we can create it *de novo* or from scratch, thus, we can function without consuming any of it. Unfortunately, we generally consume more of this least essential macronutrient that superlatively lead to insulin spike, thus making this the top offender in jeopardizing fat loss.

Proteins on the other hand, commonly come from the meaty and beefy food sources. This would include all lean meat of fish, pork, beef, chicken, white part of eggs and most beans and nuts. Its basic component is **Amino Acid.** This equates to **Grow** in the food pyramid. Some proteins can be converted to glucose, and if consumed in excess, can also lead to fat stores. Most amino acids are recyclable and can be made by our own cells. However, there are essential amino acids that need to be consumed from food since we do not have the enzymes or equipment in our cells to produce them *de novo.* To some extent, proteins also increase insulin release. And the more protein you consume, the more insulin is secreted, the more fats you store.

Once you reached adulthood, our need for protein is actually less as compared to growing children. With moderate physical activity, we require an average of 1 gram of protein per kilogram of body weight. Simply put, if you are a 70-kilogram man with an average lifestyle, you should only consume approximately 70 grams of protein in a day. This is equivalent to only about one and half matchbox size of lean meat.

This metabolic equivalent usually comes as a huge surprise for many. But this is also the reason why those who are on high-protein diet without engaging in enough strenuous physical activity leading to massive muscle breakdown are continuously gaining extra weight in the form of fats, overtime. Thus, to maintain low insulin levels, protein consumption should also be regulated.

Lastly, **Fats**. These are complex molecules that are generally oily, also known as lipids. Among the three macros, fats are the most underrated, confused and wrongly accused. Popularly known to cause heart problems and complications, fats are actually what can sustain life during prolonged fasting in the form of **ketones** as a fuel source. Note that fats are not converted to glucose or proteins, and pure natural fats are not efficient stimulus for insulin secretion, making this the most fat-loss friendly macro. Common forms of fats include lard, cooking oil, butter, egg yolk, fats from animal products and full cream dairies. It is also the basic fuel source for our heart in the form of triglycerides. And yes, it is the basic fact as to why we are informed that we have to do our cardio exercises if we want to lose the fats that are circulating in our blood stream.

Not known to all, fats is actually part of the **Go** in our food chart. It becomes an energy fuel in the form of ketones once metabolized, is a very efficient energy source not just for the heart but also for the brain and majority of the processes in our body. Like proteins, there is also what we call *essential fats*. These are the kind of fats that must be taken externally in order for our body to function properly. If consumed exclusively in our diet, or in high quantity in proportion to small part of proteins and carbohydrates, insulin spike becomes less likely, which also means that fat-storing mechanism is also on hold, and weight gain now is at minimum, if none at all.

Fat intake only becomes a problem if it is consumed together with ample amount of carbohydrates and proteins. This meal ratio will facilitate energy consumption from the easily dispensable glucose and proteins, which leads to increased insulin secretions. This increased insulin secretion will not burn the fats as energy but store it in your body in many forms. It can be stored in your liver (thus causing fatty liver), as peripheral fats (like in your thighs and arms), visceral fats (the one dangerously covering your internal organs, intestines, heart, etc.) or worse, as a bad cholesterol circulating your blood stream.

The latter form of fats are the free fats in our vascular system known as LDL (low density lipoprotein), are the ones causing problems like hypertension, heart attack and stroke. However, if fat intake is not paired with insulin-spiking foods, then, the fats you consume will be utilized as energy and will not be stored the way it could have been if insulin is also high.

Another important aspect that we need to recognize is the fact that carbohydrates do not trigger the satiety center in our brain. Meaning, it will not make you feel full/satisfied or that you've had enough. Instead, you keep on eating and eating until you feel that you are about to throw up or your stomach about to burst. You feel full but that sense of fullness is not the same sense of fullness you get by eating an avocado with slices of bacons and egg. It is because the satiety center in the brain is activated by proteins and fats, and not by carbohydrates.

Thus, if you are keen enough, you will notice that following a full meal, you can no longer take another tenderloin steak, but you can still accommodate a slice of cake. The carbohydrates from cake will not communicate your fullness to your brain hence; it is negated as far as your fullness signal is concerned. Thus, this is another reason why carbohydrate intake, especially in the form of simple sugar must be taken with utmost care. Your brain may not recognize it, but you yourself should take heed and do what is needed.

Glow foods on the other hand can be found incorporated within those three macros. These are micronutrients we need in minuscule amounts in order for all the biochemical processes in our body to go smoothly. Below is the list of vitamins and minerals we need in our daily lives. Thus, if there is a kind of food you want to eat, you make sure it has less sugar and is loaded with these nutrients since overtime, especially after fasting, these micronutrients should be replenished.

CHAPTER 11
When & How to
Break a Fast

"Fasting is the first principle of medicine. Fast and see the strength of the spirit reveal itself."

-Rumi

Engaging in fasting, especially extended ones, puts your gastrointestinal system in a temporary phase of relaxation. While the rest of your body might be active from the influx of energy from ketones, your gut is simply enjoying the calm that absence of food intake brings.

The moment you are adapted to fasting, your body simply goes on getting used to ketones as fuel source. By essence, the only essential part of our body that are made of fats are our brain and nerves, which is only about 2% of our overall body composition in males and about 10% in females (which have more necessary fats for reproductive purposes). Thus, theoretically speaking, in general, as long as our body fat percentage does not go down below 5% in men and 12% in women, we can continue to live on a fasted state while consuming only electrolytes and other essential vitamins and minerals listed in the previous chapter, as did the research volunteer who fasted for the all-time record of 382 days.

Yet, realistically speaking, it is not just practical to fast all at once until you lose all the excess fats and reach your ideal weight.

In the course of this journey, there will be a lot of times when you will be breaking your fast and it is important know when and how to properly do so. By experience, when to break a fast is largely a case to case determination.

Some fasting experts say that the return of hunger after days of loss of appetite serves as a good signal to break a fast. But personally, I consider this very subjective. Knowing that appetite can be stimulated by mere sight or smell of food, return of hunger may actually just be a physiologic manifestation of a psychological response to external factors like an advertisement of a fast food chain or the scent of your favorite meal.

If you want to be very objective about it like I do, you can monitor your body fat percentage on a daily basis while following an EF protocol. There are a number of body fat counter caliper available for sale and some calculator are incorporated in more sophisticated weighing scale. Those who don't have it can manually compute for it through various means. This website can help you with this if you are interested:

As a rule, you lose about half pound of pure body fats per 24 hours of fasting. And as long as you are doing generally well with fasting, and is not nearing the critical body fat percentage, you can continue to do so as you wish. You can then intentionally break your fast when you finally reach your goal, whether that is a goal weight, body image, percent body fat or even goal activities (that includes things you always wanted to do but cannot do so because of the extra pounds). But other than that, a good enough reason for me to break a fast is being contented with the progress I have made so far, being fulfilled with the accomplishment of completing a planned fast, and a conscious decision to go back to the dining table and enjoy the food in the company of people that I love spending time and celebrating life with. And once I decided when I will break my fast, the next thing I do is plan on how I will do it.

In fasting and in most life's undertakings, it is true what the song advocates, if you have to break it, break it gently. In general, the longer you fast, the gentler you should be in re-introducing food into your system.

After your last intended day of fasting, you can slowly consume light calorie-containing food like a vegetable soup. Since your insulin level at this point is at all-time low, your body has become more sensitive to anything that can increase your insulin, thus it is best to avoid simple, processed/refined sugars. Foods with very strong flavors or with dense composition like lean meat are better reserved the third to fourth meal after fasting as this can cause indigestion since you gut has been inactive for so long and should not be forced to function sully all at once.

There are many ways to break a fast. By thoroughly planning your fasting days until you break it, you will have a smoother transition during your period of "re-feeding" and you will have less chances of having a *"re-feeding syndrome"* wherein abrupt ending of an extended fast followed by a very heavy meal results to a medical emergency that results from sudden changes of electrolytes in a previously malnourished individual. The chances of this incidence occurring is very low especially when you follow clean fasting with basic electrolyte supplementation and is not extending this for months, but it is still a risk I do not approve for anyone to be taking.

Personally, after a 7-day fast, I recommend breaking it with one bowl of soup at the first hour and followed by a light meal 1-2 hours after. Close your window after another 2 hours with another light meal. The following day, you can proceed with your preferred maintenance IF schedule.

Remember that when fasting, your body is most sensitive to insulin after being absent for a long time. Thus, if you consume sugary foods immediately after a long fast, you are endangering your cells to its massive effects like flooding influx of glucose. Some even faint or feels light-headed after engorging a heavy meal as a "breakfast". Thus, it is very important to slowly introduce food again after a fast.

To know more about *re-feeding syndrome* and other ways to break a fast, you can check the reference for further readings.

CHAPTER 12

Foods That Enhance Fat Loss

"The philosophy of fasting calls upon us to know ourselves, to master ourselves, and to discipline ourselves the better to free ourselves."

-Tariq Ramadan

As what we previously discussed, carbohydrates and in some extent proteins, are the main cause of spikes in insulin, which eventually leads to fat storing mechanism and eventually weight gain.

Unfortunately, the danger of overconsumption of those macros doesn't stop there. Continuous influx of carbs leads to fat cells becoming *insulin* and *leptin-resistant*. With that kind of hormonal resistance, your body won't be able to know when you had enough. It is a vicious cycle where you keep on eating all those foods, storing them as fats, yet no signal on your brain that you are already full and satisfied. As a result, complications of elevated blood sugar occur. Fats that can no longer be deposited on your arms and legs are now circulating your blood stream. That bad cholesterol that freely circulates your system will eventually clog your arteries leading to high blood pressure, heart attack or stroke.

Thus, if you want to maintain fat loss during your eating window, you must seriously consider a low carbohydrate, minimal protein and high fat diet.

Out of hundreds of diet fads out there that may seem to be contradicting with each other, a common theme of foods are actually binding all of them. In general:

1. Eat whole foods. Eat only the edible foods you know were picked or harvested from plants that grew from soil or meat that previously walked or flew or swam. The more you eat them in their natural (and sanitary) state, the better. Yes, all raw edibles you can think of that can be

made into a salad are the best ones.

2. Eat less processed foods. As a rule, avoid everything that comes in packaging except for pure coconut oil for cooking, virgin olive oil consumed uncooked, real butter, full fat dairy products, and real egg-yolk mayonnaise if you cannot make it yourself (yes, you can come up with a do-it-yourself-mayonnaise). In general, I try to stick to a single-step food processing rule, that is, will eat only those that were processed once, like a grilled pork belly or fried chicken. Sparingly, I

accommodate two-step processed foods like a (1) cooked (2) honey-cured bacon. And because I am a mere fallible mortal, I allow for three- or more-step processed foods as occasional treats (i.e. cake, pastry or ice cream).

3. No simple sugar on a regular basis. Avoid as much as you can all types of table sugar, bread, pastries, cakes, potatoes especially ready-to-cook mashed ones, sodas and flavored drinks, beer and flavored alcoholic drinks,

4.   Think of portions when you eat. Not in quantity but in quality. In general, you can fill up one large plate with high fiber, low carbohydrate veggies, and another smaller plate with some proteins like eggs and something sumptuous like pork steak. Isn't that mouth-watering?

See below the green list on the food you can eat that can still help weight loss even when eaten until satisfaction. The suggested ratio of a maximum of 20 grams carbohydrates (see options below), 1 gram/kg of bodyweight of protein (no more than 100 grams) and 70-80% of calories from natural fats per day. (*see appendix* B)

Note that by eating a low carbohydrate, high fat diet, or *a Ketogenic Diet*, will biochemically mimic ketosis, thus will put you in a state similar to that when one is engaging in prolonged fasting despite only doing IF.

Approved Green List of Foods You Can Eat Freely

1. **Carbohydrates** – must contain 0-5 grams of net carbohydrates per 100 grams, eaten fresh, cooked or fermented like kimchi or pickled as long as there is no added sugar.

a. All green leafy vegetables like spinach, cabbage, brussel sprouts, malunggay, lettuce, sweet potato leves, kangkong and many more.

b. Low-carbohydrate vegetables – cauliflower, broccoli, bell peppers, asparagus, cucumber, zucchini, celery, radishes

c. Fruits – generally all fruits are high in carbohydrate content, portions of berries, watermelon, cantaloupe, avocado, honeydew, peaches and mature coconut meat may be eaten when a "dessert" is necessary.

2. Proteins – proteins should be kept below 1 gram per kilogram of body per day to avoid excessive glucose conversion through gluconeogenesis. For example, a 70-kg man should limit protein intake to only 70 grams, or about 1.5 palm size of meat per day. Overeating should be avoided. The following are the common sources of proteins you can choose from:

   a. Animal Proteins - All meats and meat products cure in natural processes including sausages and salami, eggs, offal/internal organs and Seafood except Sword Fish and tilefish due to high mercury content

b. Plant-based proteins – most nuts in limited amount (almonds, peanuts, flaxseed, chia, macadamia, pecan, pumpkin, sunflower seeds, walnut), mushrooms, and beans

3. Fats – healthy, natural fats should be the primary source of energy or daily caloric requirements. Although you can generally eat all that you want, make sure that you only eat when you are hungry and

stop eating as soon as you are full or satisfied. Avoid eating sweet foods to counter the feelings of being "fed up". Instead, listen to your body and just stop eating because it's a good signal that you've really had enough. Although you would still be in ketosis if you eat more that what you will need, however, your body will burn the energy coming from the fats you consume and not the extra fats stored in your body. Here are the list of healthy fats you take during your window:

a. Plant-based – Avocado oil, coconut milk and oil, olives and olive oil, macadamia oil

b. Animal-based – All full-cream dairy products, soft and hard cheeses, yogurt, egg yolk, cream, creamcheese, all types of animal fat from beef, pork, chicken, duck or salmon, butter, ghee, duck fat, butter and full-fat mayonnaise.

4. Other food products

   a. Any condiments and seasonings without added sugar, preservatives and vegetable oil like pepper, cinnamon, cayenne powder and many more.

   b. Sweeteners – ideally should be avoided as this still cause insulin spike despite low sugar content, but when necessary, opt for the following: erythritol granules, stevia leaves/powders, xylitol granules, and monk fruit.

CHAPTER 13
Foods to Avoid to Ensure Fat Loss

"Start the practice of self-control with penance; begin with fasting."

-Mahavira

As you can see, the worst type of food when in the process of fat loss are carbohydrates and in some extent, over eating of proteins.

However, you might think that taking away carbs, also means, taking away your joy. Don't be overdramatic; you know that is not true. With internet and thousands of food geniuses sharing their knowledge, you can practically have almost everything in low carbohydrate alternative. Don't believe me? Try Googling "Low Carb

Dinner Rolls Recipe" and you won't be missing the real thing.

You see, I believe the favorite kinds of carbs can be divided into three types: first are those that neutralize a sumptuous main course, like a mashed potato or a simple pasta, rice or bread. Secondly, there are carbohydrates that are needed because they help with bowel movement. And lastly, it makes up most of our desserts. And since we cannot completely do away with it, it is important that we try to understand carbohydrates better so we can manage our intake sparingly yet still be successful with our journey to better health.

First, let's tackle why we are so used to have something bland or less tasteful to accompany a perfectly good steak? This can be understood by examining the following major reasons:

A. Economical - It may no longer be applicable to you now, but as expenses are part of day to day, two cups of mashed potato is still cheaper than another slice of steak. Thus, with less cost, you will be "filled" faster. So, if you are actually not saving, you can do away with it. And if like me, you are also conscious with your spending, there are so many low carbohydrate alternatives that are affordable to pair with your favorite steak.

B. Too much flavor makes you feel fed-up easily - When you are eating something very delicious, like a slab of roast pork, no matter how much you like it, you can only consume up to a certain amount and you know you can no longer take another bite. Unless, you accompany it with something with lesser flavor, to "neutralize" it.

Although it is truly understandable, you have to recognize that the feeling of "fullness", satisfied and satiated even if you've just eaten less than half of what your stomach can accommodate, is a normal bodily function that we should be very sensitive about. Again, it is the fats and proteins that trigger that Satiety Center in our brain and not the carbohydrates. So if you are feeling "satiated", you can just stop eating and drink coffee, tea or water to fill up the remaining space. However, if like me, you also want the physical feeling of fullness, then I recommend you take note of the alternatives on the green list that you can eat as much as you can without worrying the carbohydrate count.

C. Carbohydrates are essential in our toilet routines - Yes; we need carbohydrates to do our favorite morning alone time. Although some experts suggest that daily bowel movement is more of a psychological routine rather than a physical need, a lot of us feel good after some bowel elimination, thus, the incorporation of some amount of carbohydrates is mostly preferred. But remember that what you need is a specific kind of carbohydrate called dietary fiber. These fibers will give bulk to your stool to eliminate wastes properly. With adequate water intake, your toilet moments will still go smoothly so long as you consume a low carbohydrate, high fiber meals. (*see the vegetable options in the green list*)

Lastly, who can live without desserts? Surely I can't. Although during the first few months I completely eradicated all the sweets I´ve known my whole life. I decided to enroll myself in a self-imposed "Sugar Addiction Rehabilitation", and I believe I succeeded for 2 straight months. After, I then slowly reintroduced sweets in our kitchen with the good kind. And this time, with control. I make large batches of low-carb fat bombs and chocolate puddings and amazingly almost never touch them in my fridge. I tricked my brain with the idea that I have ample supply of sweets that I can go to anytime, and with that, my interest just die down.

As a rule, I do not use simple sugars. As an alternative, I use Stevia or

Monkfruit sweetener, these are natural, organic, low to zero calorie sweetener you can use with caution. And since they cost more than table sugar, and still stimulate the same pleasure center in our brain and to some extent elevate insulin despite being zero-calorie content, I use them at minimum and the final dessert; I eat only when I have cravings that now occur very rarely.

For further guidance, see the Unapproved Red List below on foods that can jeopardize your journey towards ideal body weight. In general, these are processed foods, sugary, artificial, some whole but carbo-loaded foods like pasta, rice, noodles, potatoes, cereals and even most fruits. Also, for best outcome, kindly avoid cigarette smoking and alcohol consumption in addition to food that you eat during an open window until our two months target is reached.

Note that when one is still on the process of losing weight, EF is recommended. But if only IF is feasible, then it is strongly suggested to do it with the right foods and avoid all that's in the red list as possible. This way, you will be able to see results as if you are engaging in EF as well.

Unapproved Red List Foods to be Avoided

In general, these food options are not essential for your survival. It may activate the pleasure center in your brain (*the same center triggered by illicit drugs like cocaine*) and subsequently, sugar addiction, but it will do nothing good in your journey towards reaching your health goal. These may be eaten in very rare occasions, and in portions but never a weekly or even monthly routine.

1. Traditional baked products – any food products containing flours, corn, wheat, rice, cassava, potato or other starchy foods. These include bread, cookies, and pastries.

2. All artificial drinks and fruits juices as these contain mostly either of corn syrup, high amounts of fructose or artificial sweeteners.

3. Processed dairy products, cheese spreads, coffee creamers, condensed milk, icecreams, rice and soy milk and anything fat-free or low-fat counterpart.

4. Toxic, processed fats like regular chocolates, seed oils, sunflower, vegetable and canola oils, commercially prepared chocolate bars, syrups and related products, commercial sauces, margarines and most prepared salad dressings.

5. Fruits and vegetables – most fruits and vegetables not mentioned above are either high in sugar or fructose, refined carbohydrates of high calorie from starch like peas, potatoes, beetroots, cassava, and excessive amount of peanuts and legumes.

6. Meat- 'unfermented soy or vegetarian proteins, meats cured mostly in sugar and other highly processed meat products like canned meats, sausages and meat loafs.

7. Sweeteners – all forms of sugar in various names like table sugar, brown, white, muscovado, coco sugar, artificial sweeteners, dried

fruits, fructose, honey, candies, syrups and commercially prepared flavorings of any kind.

8. General – all fast foods because they usually use vegetable oils for frying and processed meats and high carbohydrate products, all processed foots, and any food with added sugar.

CHAPTER 14
No Cheating, Make Plans Instead

"Fasting is necessary as feasting."

-Laila Gifty Akita

Celebrations are part of any social culture. And this lifestyle doesn't prohibit you from enjoying and indulging whenever the situation calls for it.

Single day celebrations like birthdays, weddings and anniversaries don't need much adjustment. You can simply extend your fast the day before or after to fit the schedule. Note though that *Sunday Family Day*, as it occurs weekly, is no more special than Mondays or Wednesdays. Should you decide to indulge weekly, you might as well consider doing an extended fast each day after as well, just enough to burn all the extra calories you've taken. That's the beauty of this lifestyle, you can design it in your own personal way with the knowledge in mind of how our body works and what fuel it burns depending on how long have you fasted and what you've been consuming prior to fasting. This way, it's almost like it never happened.

The challenge usually comes on longer celebratory days like Christmas Season that extend to new year, or a long thanksgiving week, or the vacation cruise you have been planning for years. The dictum on this would be the following:

1. Enjoy the best way you can while considering food as a minor source of happiness. If unable to do so, consider #2.

2. Try doing at least 16 hours fasting. Breakfast buffets usually last until 10 in the morning while dinner can start as early as 5PM and you can end it by 6PM.

3. Try sticking to ketogenic food choices, or at least have whole foods if avoidance already jeopardizes your happiness.

4. If all else fails, just enjoy the whole length and just get back to your routine as soon as your vacation is over. Since this is a lifestyle, you have to go back to your normal, that is, a combination of fasting and Low Carb High Fat (LCHF) eating pattern. Sure you would gain some pounds, but you will take it off in no time.

In order for you to avoid the feeling of guilt, plan your days ahead. Avoid using the term cheat day as this denotes dishonesty, something that is opposite to what we are aiming here. Instead, do some planned indulgences, where you will give in to foods and timing that is out of your routine for something special. This way, you will be able to have a harmonious relationship with food and you make sure you enjoy every bite and moments you share it with.

CHAPTER 15
What about Exercise?

"The goal of fasting is inner unity."

-Thomas Merton

By now you probably have the idea why exercise is not really essential for weight loss. While it is true that the more energy you spend on exercising means the more calories you burn, the net effect may not necessarily be weight loss. As you know, a lot of factors are in place.

During an exercise routine, your body will consume energy similar to that when you are fasting. However, as you exercise, your metabolic rate or the amount of energy needed for you to function also increases. This phenomenon, paired with depletion of electrolytes and muscle fatigue will lead to increased demand for food. Hunger hormone *Ghrelin* will soar up high. Failure to deny what your body is craving will only lead to a rebound effect of consuming more than what you just probably need. And of course, we all know where that road leads.

In addition, studies show that extreme and strenuous exercises doesn't equate to sustained increase in metabolism simply because our body adapts to it and our metabolism plateaus despite increased physical activity. Thus, it is another factor why it does not follow that the more you exercise, the more you lose weight, as seen in the famous television show, the biggest loser, or anybody you know who lost weight initially after going the gym but gained it back or plateaued eventually.

But with proper mindset and just the right amount of time and moderate intensity, exercise can actually boost weight loss effect in terms of fat stores. Wonder why I mentioned fat stores? It is because exercise can increase muscle bulk, and muscle weighs heavier than fats! That is why weight is actually not the best gauge for good health

But if we are honest enough with ourselves, you know for sure whether what you have are muscles buried under the fats, or just fats above a thin muscle.

In addition, studies show that the more you exercise, doesn't really lead to more fat loss from increased metabolism. This is because our body adapts to it, a.k.a. *metabolic adaptation,* thus making it less and less efficient as you increase your physical activities to the extreme.

Don't get me wrong, I am not saying that you should not exercise because we know that exercise have numerous advantages like brain plasticity, endurance, and improved sense of well-being, body contouring, physical strength and even some degree of anti-aging effects. These benefits can be attained just by having moderate exercise activity like running for 30 minutes five times a week. But when it comes to weight loss, exercise is simply not required especially if you don't want to.

CHAPTER 16
Weight Loss Plateau

"Fasting is not just a spiritual discipline; it can be a spiritual feast."

-Jentezen Franklin

When this occurs, ask yourself first if you really need to lose more weight or if you are already enjoying your weight goal? How long have you been in this lifestyle? Have you been following a strict LCHF meal plans? Are you religious in sticking to your fasting schedule? Be honest with yourself and re-assess how you can improve your routine by starting again. Do not hurry and trust the process. Give it at least two full months before you jump into sad conclusions. Because there are some who started with slow metabolism from a previous low calorie diet and may even experience weight gain during the first few weeks when the body is still adjusting. Always remember that this lifestyle is not about perfection but continued improvement. The progress that you do in making better choices each day and the commitment to get back on track as soon as you realize you unintentionally fell off the wagon is always an achievement in itself. You sticking to this lifestyle even after achieving your goal signify self-love. However, despite doing everything right and the weight loss plateaus, you may consider the following options

1. Level up your fasting schedule. If you've been having IF or 24H fasting, you can increase it one level higher or try doing a minimum of 3 days extended fast. If you are not yet in your ideal goal, then there is no plateauing in extended fasting. Just make sure you are not underweight and your body fat percentage does not go below 10-12% which is considered the minimum with a safety net before you jeopardize neurological processes in your body.

2.   Try doing a *fat fast* for five days. This schedule is advocated by Dr. Atkin. In this protocol, you fast for 5 days, but each day, you can have 5 small all-fat intakes in a 5-hour eating period. Examples of fats you can consume are cream cheese with some cocoa or peanut butter, full fat heavy cream, MCT oil, grass-fed butter, full fat mayonnaise and coconut cream. Consume no more than 250 kcal of fat each time.

3.   Check your meals, because even if you are doing LCHF, you might have overlooked your protein consumption. Know that

you only need minimal protein intake even for when you are working out. The muscle breakdown that happens during exercise is very minimal and the necessary proteins for repair and bulk formation can be obtained from the process of *autophagy*.

4. Do some measurements. For all you know, your body is reshaping. With *autophagy* that occurs especially when you are engaging in 24-hour fast or more, the fats are reduced and the muscles increase in the right places. And since muscles weigh more than fats, you might actually be really losing fats and

gaining more muscles. This is the reason why I advocate doing measurements like your arms, waist, hips and neck circumference before starting anything. A mirror selfie on front, side and back also provides a very good gauge, and oftentimes better than the scale.

5. Check with your physician if you have other hormonal imbalance that could possibly lead to weight gain like *hypothyroidism* or *hyperaldosteronism* or *hyperinsulinemia*. Although these conditions can actually benefit from this lifestyle,

certain conditions might need proper investigation in order for it to be properly managed medically.

6. Check your prescriptions and ask your doctor if weight gain is a part of the side effects. If so, you can try asking if you can be slowly weaned from it (since fasting actually helps your body heal naturally) or change it for an alternative.

7. Double check your food portions. Although doing *fasting* boosts metabolism through increased adrenaline, after significant weight loss,

especially drastic ones, your metabolism sometimes slows down. For others who started with slower metabolism, you might initially need to cut back a part of what you are consuming and follow an OMAD lifestyle for at least two months. With this, your metabolism will normalize and as you become sensitive with your body, you will only eat when you really need to and stop when you are satisfied.

With these in mind, you can always have a back-up plan, whenever you hit a bump along the way. Trust that it is possible. Trust that it is a proven science. Trust that you can do it and remember how badly you want it in the first place.

CHAPTER 17
Why & How I Started Fasting

"Fasting is futile unless it is accompanied by an incessant longing for self-restraint."

-Mahatma Gandhi

Growing up, I have always felt that the way I look is not who I am inside. Despite reassurance from other people that I look and weighed "okay", a part of me always knew that I can do better, that I can be better. And it is only later that I realized that the physical improvement was just secondary, but how I healed myself psychologically, through discipline, self-control and fasting, made all the difference.

I had asthma as a child and was diagnosed with allergic *rhinoconjunctivitis* during the later years. All my unfiltered pictures always show my *allergic shiners*, these are the dark circles around the eyes typical of people suffering from chronic inflammation and allergies. I have been maintaining an intranasal steroid and oral antihistamines for my allergies.

[*You know I once kid my friend that I am allergic to everything. And she said, that is impossible or else I'd be dead. I told her I am primarily allergic to make-up and dogs, and that's practically everything. But seriously, my allergies already affected my everyday life.*]

Because of my height, I was always recruited on different sports like basketball, soccer, lawn tennis, badminton, volleyball and even table tennis, and I engaged whenever the opportunity arise. But off intramural season, I would rather choose to be still, eat, sleep and enjoy the afternoon with my loved ones. As a result, I never really developed any muscles. And soon I realized I have water retention where my lower body becomes edematous later during the day. As a doctor, I know I only need to exercise to strengthen the muscles on my lower legs and improve my overall circulation. But, I always find a good excuse not to exercise. One of my favorite excuses would be the idea that I am trying to live a minimalistic life, thus, doing physical exertion without actual work accomplishment in the form of exercise just doesn't seem to fit. Plus, I feel much better after a nap than anything.

Other than that, I feel like I am where I am supposed to be, from career, relationship, personal development and family. Food is the only aspect of my life that I am not in control with. Thus, I have decided that if I can gain control over food, I can gain control with any other aspects of my life.

I then began researching until I learned about fasting. And the benefits it comes with. Upon knowing the wide array of advantages from fasting, I decided I will do it for physical, mental and spiritual purposes. Together with my family, we embarked on a 5-day water-only fast, with some apple cider vinegar for potassium and salt water for sodium. We went about our normal day with our usual tasks and we succeeded with ease. We all lost a good amount of fats and the most dramatic would be the reversal of *hypertriglyceridemia* (from more than 2500 down to only 230 after a month) on one of us. Over time, we engaged in intermittent fasting and occasionally extending our fast. I lost a total of about 22-25 pounds and I am now at an all-time sustained low weight of 115 pounds and I never felt any better. During active fasting, I have been at my lowest of 108 pounds to which I easily gained the water loss after.

Aside from being very comfortable with my own body now, I also get a lot of compliments that I look a lot younger, possibly with my skin. And most importantly, I never get the need for antihistamine and intranasal steroids. My allergies are the things of the past and I can easily hug my dogs and put make-up without experiencing any itch.

I shared what I learned with the people closest to my heart and I am so happy that they too have started on this journey. I have people who are closest to me and grew up with that used to be overweight and now has normal BMI. There is another that is from size 6 to size 0, and one with a lifetime of acne problems and with smoother skin. From diabetes and hypertension to no medication needed. And from uncomfortable, to now being happy in his own skin. Like them, I want you to be free too, free from food, free from being branded as the fat one, free from the stigma that you will never have the chance to have that perfect body you so aim to have. If my story isn't enough, you can find a lot of testimonials and stories from real people online. You will know for sure that it is no fad since nobody else can have an ulterior motive with you being at your healthiest. The main beneficiary is just you, plainly and exclusively you.

If somebody told me that I can achieve the weight that I have now in a month's time before, there's no way I would ever believe. The BMI and weight that I have now is something I never dreamed of because I never thought it is possible. But it is, and I have never felt better and comfortable in my own skin than now. Finally, the way I looked, the way I see myself in the mirror, is already the person that I always felt to be inside.

It may be faster or slower with you, but trust that in time, you will have it too.

In summary, this is what I did chronological order:

1. Five days of water-only fast, with apple cider vinegar a salt (lost 10 lbs)

2. Two weeks of approximately 16:8 clean IF, no

simple sugars (kept 6 lbs of the weight loss)

3. 10.5 days water-only fast (lost another 15 lbs)

4. Two weeks of 16 to 24-hour clean fast (maintained the ~20 lbs weight loss, already on goal of 19-20 BMI score)

5. Seven days water-only fast - (lost another 5lbs but gained back after a feast from a week-long vacation)

6. Maintenance of 19 to 20 hours IF/OMAD lifestyle, trying my best to stick to a low-carb but with occasional moderate to high carb intake. Incorporation

of 24-36 hour fast after a feast or whenever I have a high-carb intake.

From a previously impaired fasting blood glucose level of 110-115 mg/dL, it is now down to 79 mg/dL and an HbA1c of 5.3% (diabetes cut off is 6.5%).

IF is now my way of life as I have reached my target weight. I do cyclical EF for other purposes (*autophagy, anti-aging and immune boosting effects whenever I have flu*). I still do not have a regular physical activity but I also do not avoid long walks, stairs and far parking lots. Overall, I feel like my best version

yet and there is nothing I wish for you
than to be the best version of you too.
☺

CHAPTER 18
Motivational Thoughts and Tips During Fasting

- First, believe.

- If others can do it, I can too.

- All good food can wait.

- A large group of people worldwide are into fasting, be it for religious, health or philosophical reasons.

- This may not be important to you, but even celebrities swear by it including *Hugh Jackman, Beyonce, Jennifer Lopez, Nicole Kidman, Benedict Cumberbatch, Ben Affleck* and many more. https://www.delish.com/food/g2 2617665/celebrities-intermittent-fasting/

- Before eating out of your window, ask yourself, is this a

nutritional eating or just an emotional eating?

- Always remember what certain foods make you feel. (*Like for me, eating sugary foods reactivates my allergic rhinoconjunctivitis. It gives me itchy eyes as well as bloated stomach and return of cravings, making fasting hours even more difficult.*)

- Don't compare yourself with other's weight loss pace. Compare yourself with your previous self. Even if you are not losing as much, be glad that as of this moment, you are no longer gaining more weight.

- As they say, just mind your own plate.

- Fasting and eating healthy has multitude of benefits that goes beyond weight loss.

- This is not a quick fix diet this is a lifestyle that is sustainable as a permanent way of life.

- Once you have done an extended fast, missing a meal or two or even a day becomes no big deal.

- Fasting makes eating pleasurable by a hundred fold. A meal becomes not just a meal but a celebration of life. If you engage in OMAD, imagine a feeling of happiness and celebration each and every day.

- When fasting, you become much focused and your attention to detail accelerates.

- Eating sweet foods, even artificial sweetener spikes insulin and reactivates sugar addiction for those affected. Thus, it is a big No-no during fasting and must be done with caution during your eating window.

- Do not jeopardize what you have done just because you felt emotional and needed food. Try drinking water first and go for a 10 minute walk with fresh air and see how it works.

- Fasting allows you to do guilt-free feasting on momentous occasions with loved ones.

- Only you have the power to give this gift to yourself.

- Physical appearance is not everything that matters, but, our own personal image about how we see ourselves does.

- Let your self be the representative of the real and ideal you.

- Discipline is a state of mind.

- Fasting is 95% psychological challenge.

- Practice your mental strength through fasting and by saying no to unhealthy foods.

- The primary person who can benefit from all these is you.

- Never stop believing, you can do it.

- Give it at least 2 strict months before giving up totally.

- What is two months as compared to a life-long benefit?

- How do you feel about reversing signs of aging through fasting?

- With proper guidance, how do you feel about the possibility of not needing maintenance medications anymore for allergies, asthma, diabetes, high cholesterol and hypertension?

- When you are fasting, you are in a protective and conservative mode. Your immune system is heightened, thus, protecting you from common illnesses like flu and cold.

- I fast to heal my body.

- I fast to improve my mind.

- I fast for clarity and focus.

- I fast for ideas.

- Fasting is being efficient, that includes no spending for extra food while I still have fats to burn.

- The moment I eat, I become relaxed and instantly lose the critical thinking I had moments before I give in to food.

- I can delay eating a certain food if my window is not yet open. But I can remember how it tastes like simply because the foods that I like are the foods I have eaten many times before. The memory of its taste will be enough until my window opens.

- And yes, you too can wait until your window opens.

- Weight is only a small aspect of fasting. Do not be a slave of the weighing scale. Your body is likely reshaping and improving more than the scale can tell.

- Try to move from the scale until you finish the minimum two months cycle.

- When fasting, your work productivity increases.

- Do not be discouraged when the scale doesn't seem to move as much as you want it to. Trust the process and for some it takes time.

- Have other gauge of improvement aside from scale like, a monthly mirror photo, how "honesty" pants/clothes fit, *how light you feel,* how radiant your skin has become and how others keep on commenting you are slimming down.

- Do not mind others who are discouraging you from not eating. They were not there when you were eating unhealthy foods 6 times a day.

- If others are giving negative comments about your practice and how you look "so skinny", try to assess first if there is genuine concern from that person or just an uneducated opinion. Otherwise, if you see you are still on your healthy range of BMI and are functioning well, you are good to go.

- This is your own journey. If others will join, then well and good, but if there is no one else in your circle, keep on and remember that there is so much strength and reward in going and achieving solo.

- Be patient.

- A common reason for fasting failure is boredom and subsequent preoccupation with food. Be prepared and be productive. Plan your days ahead, best by doing something worthwhile or even by just binge-watching a very good TV series.

- Join various support groups in social media, just type in keywords like extended fasting, intermittent fasting or one meal a day.

- Download an app that tracks your daily fasting goals.

- Reward yourself with non-food trophies after a successful fast or after achieving a certain goal.

- Keep yourself busy during a planned fast.

- Plan a productive activity during EF.

- Strive for continued improvement, and not perfection.

- Be kind to yourself.

- If all else fails, send me a message and I'd be very happy to help. My email is <u>josephinegracechuarojo@gmail.com</u>

CHAPTER 19
Other Benefits of Fasting

"I fast for greater physical and mental efficiency."

-Plato

It is said that weight loss is only a side effect of fasting, although a beneficial one at that. However, the real benefit of fasting is said to occur not in the visible scale but in more significant and qualitative way. The following are the good effects of fasting in our health:

- Reduces risk of developing cancer and even shrinks certain tumors.

- Decreases allergic and inflammatory diseases such as

allergic rhinitis, arthritis, joint pains, and even asthma.

- Unbelievable as it may seem, but when done right, fasting gives more energy and stamina to do heavier work.

- Reverses type II diabetes in select patients

- Normalizes blood pressure for those with essential hypertension.

- Clears and heals skin diseases like acne and eczema.

- Normalizes ovulation especially for women suffering from polycystic ovarian syndrome.

- Decreases bad cholesterol level and reduces arterial occlusion thereby decreasing risk for stroke and heart attack.

- Slows aging and promotes longevity through autophagy.

- Improves neurologic functioning.

- Decreases risk for developing neurodegenerative diseases such as *Alzheimer 's disease*.

The details of each benefit and how to go about it is already beyond the scope of this book. It is included in the succeeding books of this series. Meantime, I believe that it is of great importance that we are all aware of such benefits. Now that you are knowledgeable with the basics of fasting and how it can improve our way of life, I encourage you to do your own readings and research so we can educate many more, especially those near our hearts, and so we can get more out of this life TOGETHER.

CHAPTER 20
Summary and Pearls

"Fasting of the body is food for the soul."

-Saint John Chrysostom

Problem with weight management is not something that occurred overnight. One cannot simply blame their own eating habits because it goes back more than that. In fact, it is only a manifestation of an underlying erroneous way of dealing with food that goes back for centuries already.

Like it or not, we are all a byproduct of upbringing by multi-billion food industry that influenced our parents and grandparents to an eating pattern that actually unnatural to humans. As our genetic make-up is still like that of our hunter-gatherer ancestors, we have to embrace and incorporate fasting as our way of life. Without it, our body will keep on storing body fats until it can no longer accommodate it in its limited compartment and eventually disrupt our body's balance. This disturbance in our metabolic homeostasis can then manifest as obesity, high blood pressure, diabetes, fatty liver, rapid aging, tumors and even death from stroke and heart attack. Thus, in order to start the healing process, we should strive to eliminate first the excess fat stores that we have and allow our body to refocus its energy in order for it to repair itself. This is facilitated by fasting. Doing so will allow us to slowly burn the excess fats that we have been storing our whole life. Through, extended fasting, one can safely achieve an ideal weight the shortest possible time. I personally believed that a 7-day clean extended fast (EF) can be done and in the words of my editor, *"it is either to go big or go home"*. However, I truly respect individual differences as well as preferences. I am pro-choice after all. So for those who are more comfortable with the *"slowly but surely process"*, intermittent fasting (IF) is the next best thing. Both fasting schedule can lead to **ketosis**, which is the fat-burning mode of our body and our aim in achieving in our goal to an efficient weight loss process. In addition, we also identify clean fasting versus dirty fasting, wherein, if you choose to engage in a clean fast, you are only allowed to consume water, black coffee, plain tea leaves, vinegar and pure electrolytes like salt. Note that the only way to go with IF is through a clean fast. However, when you decide to do an extended fast, you can have more liberty in your fluids should you decide to do an EF through dirty *fasting*. To recap, here's the difference between the following:

- Extended fasting – fasting for 24 hours of more. I advocate for everyone to try to engage in a 5-

7 days EF as a jumpstart of ketosis and maintain on IF after. This will give you the most benefit in terms of weight loss, gastrointestinal system rest and a great mental booster for your future fasting schedules.

1. Clean Fasting – drink water only when feeling hungry or thirsty. You can have black coffee or plain tea. When feeling weak, take some salts by either taking it as is, or mix it in your water, black coffee, tea or some vinegar to make it more palatable. I advise that you try to do clean fasting

as long as you can. I did it for 11 days and stopped only when I already felt some cramps on my legs as I walk up in a ramp. Too bad, I didn't have magnesium supplements that time counter it. But should you plan to do it more than 7 days, I suggest that you will do it prepared. Kindly refer back to chapter 5 for a full list of electrolytes that u can take while on a clean fast.

2. Dirty Fasting – reserve this in times when you can no longer sustain a clean fast.

It is where you can consume calorie containing foods rich with healthy fats and nutrients that can help some sustain an EF. This would include vegetable and bone broth, MCT oil, pure coconut oil, butter, heavy whipped cream and whole full fat milk.

- Intermittent fasting – this is when you fast for less than 24 hours. It may take some time before one is fully adjusted to IF. But I find that after about three days or so of headache, weakness and extreme hunger, people who are used to breakfast generally adapts well on the fourth day and those who are used to skipping breakfast adapts more easily. A clean fast is encouraged during IF. You can slowly decrease your *"eating window"* from 12 hours to eventually 4-5 hours only eating one full meal with 1- 2 light snacks before your window closes. Remember that a bottle of beer or a glass of wine already constitutes as a light snack and should not be taken lightly.

Fasting, whether IF or EF is the core essence of managing weight. But for optimum health, it is optimum to maximize the benefits by eating the right foods when you can. The best foods to eat during a window period will actually depend from person to person. I recommend you to read Gin Stephen's book entitled *Feast Without Fear* wherein she beautifully describe the kind of foods that are best consumed by certain body types. But to be on the safe side, I believe in the science behind a Low Carbohydrate High Fat diet wherein you avoid carbo-loaded foods that are not natural to the large part of human development, like breads, pasta, mashed potato, rice and noodles, especially when you haven't reached your goal weight yet. Another set of foods you have to avoid are processed foods full of preservatives and simple sugars as in table sugar, or those incorporated in foods like in common desserts, colas, fruit juices, blended coffees and other drinks. While you are still on initial phase of trying to lose weight, it is best to avoid fruits as they are mostly full of fructose. Safe fruits would include avocado, coconut and berries. For those who have sugar addiction or are always craving for sweets and chocolates, it is a good opportunity to practice avoidance and rehabilitate your palate away from the addicting taste. However, if this is not yet your time to do so, know that there are so many easy low-carb chocolate recipes online available for free. Just ask Google. ☺

As long as you are not pregnant, breastfeeding or a growing child, you can certainly fast! For those with medical conditions, kindly ask your trusted physician for advice first prior to engaging in such.

Once you have decided to proceed with fasting, you must also know when to break it. Although it is common to overeat after a fast, it is also noticeable that those that made it into a way of life already breaks the fast slowly. And breaking the fast gently is really the way we should do it.

For special days, holidays and vacations, you can certainly enjoy these precious moments both with food and family. Weight loss plateaus or even weight gain after a weight loss should not become a concern because you already know what to do when you need to and really want to.

Trust the process and you will certainly attain the ideal weight and optimum health you've always been dreaming of.

CHAPTER 21
Frequently Asked Questions

I believe that reading the book from cover to cover will give enlightenment to common questions. And sometimes, it is good to re-read either the whole book or certain chapters after you have already adapted to fasting as a way of life. However, for any gray area that this book may have, kindly send me a personal message and I welcome it with open arms. Whether it is a suggestion, a question or a need for improvement, I consider it a pleasure and an opportunity to make this better.

This chapter will be updated from time to time. As of this writing, the following are the FAQs:

- *Is fasting the same as starving?* No, because fasting is a deliberate, conscious and unforced decision of not consuming any calorie-containing foods for a specific period of time. The person who is fasting can choose to stop it at any time he/she wishes to. It is commonly done for health, religious, and philosophical reasons.

- *When will I know that I need to take electrolytes during an extended fast?* Each electrolyte abnormality will present differently. Weakness during the early days of fasting is commonly due to sodium depletion, thus, you can take in some salt little by little not going more than 3 teaspoon per day. Whereas, cramps may mean low in magnesium on the later days. See Chapter 5 for details.

- *How will I know when I will break my fast?* Kindly go back to Chapter 11 for the specifics. However, it is best to know your health status by checking your BMI and Body Fat Percentage does not go below normal while correlating it with how your body feels. Always listen to your body and do not jeopardize anything life threatening just for the sake of weight loss. Remember that you can always fast again should you feel the need to cut a planned EF.

- Is extended *fasting* a requirement to lose weight? This depends on your goal and how would you like to go about it. If you are like me and my sister who wanted to test the waters right in, and see how we would perform, and see results significantly per day, then EF is for you. But as per weight loss per se, it is not necessary. There are numerous success stories even just with IF alone and a maintenance of OMAD after.

- *After about 2 weeks in this lifestyle, I feel light but the scale doesn't seem to move nor I look slimmer, is this okay?* Yes, it is okay. Remember that it is important to give it at least two months before you can really see substantial and visible results. However, you may in fact feel lighter because you are actually losing fats that are not visibly obvious but are very important to your health. These are visceral fats or the dangerous fats that surrounds your internal organs like your liver, heart and intestines. Thus, do not worry and fast on!

- *I tried IF before and I cannot tolerate the headache and I am afraid I might faint. Can I really do it?* If you are not part of those identified in Chapter 7, I believe you certainly can. Acknowledge that the headache and light-headedness are common side-effects of the transition from the process of sugar/glucose-burning to fat-burning state. You have the option to relax during these times for you to feel at ease, but you can also make yourself busy and preoccupied with something worthwhile to take your mind off it. Although there is in fact science behind these challenges, it also has a remedy (like electrolytes or rest). And it is not an exaggeration when we say that fasting is largely a challenge on mental strength than a physical one.

- *Why my face does looks slimmer but my stomach still looks bloated?* You may be fasting the right way, which is, getting into ketosis and fat-burning state. But it is time that you have to take a look at what you have been eating during your window. Remember, to achieve the maximum benefit, you have to pair fasting with the right healthy foods, especially whole, raw, unprocessed or least processed foods. Sugary and carbohydrate-rich foods tend to hold more water than fats and proteins. Thus, this water retention may be the cause of your persistent weight and *bloated-ness*.

- *Is it okay to overeat during my window?* Yes and no. Studies show that even if you feel like you overeat during your window, the amount you consume is still less than the amount you could have consumed if you have eaten 3 times a day on a regular breakfast-lunch-dinner routines. So, you can it is "okay", although it is not advisable to really overeat during your window. It is again important to listen more to your body and just eat until you are full and satisfied. And even if in a way it is "not okay", but it is expected during the first weeks of getting into this lifestyle, and you will just be surprised when time comes you suddenly get full even before you finish your planned feast. Overtime, I hope your feast will be trimmed down into a meal but still with the sense of satisfaction similar to that of a feast!

- *What is your recommended IF schedule?* It will depend on your goal. If you are still starting this way of life (WOL) and in the period of adjusting, I recommend you lengthen it as long as you can. From 12 hours, you can try to reach a minimum of 16-18 hours in order to have a substantial effect. Believe or not, you will soon realize that a 6-8 hours window period is just a long time to allow us to eat. You will see that food is something that takes so much energy to process and a longer fasting period means more efficient time for your body to burn what you ate and tap the fat stores you are yet to burn. As for maintenance, I personally believe in OMAD (one meal a day) that again means one full meal with 1-2 light snacks on a 4-5 hours window period. This 19-20 hours fasting period is what I recommend for those who already reached their goal weight without jeopardizing their metabolism.

- *Is exercise necessary for weight loss?* As per Chapter 15, the answer is no. But exercise is best for other reasons like building muscles, endurance and strength. The advantages are at maximum when done together with fasting and when you already achieved your target weight.

- *For females, how do you sustain fasting when you have your period?* Although female hormones are at the lowest during the menstrual period, none of it directly affects your metabolism and functioning. With adequate fluid intake and mental practice, fasting can be done safely and efficiently.

- *Can you continue working while fasting?* As I have mentioned many times, I am a doctor working in a very busy public hospital for 10-24 hours daily. I perform surgeries for 4-12 hours straight during my EFs and nobody would have believed me have they known it that time because I am functioning similarly or even better than when I was not fasting.

- *Once I achieved my target weight, can I stop fasting and go back to eating the "usual" way?* You can certainly do so. But, chances are, you will also go back to your previous body before you started it all. Thus, if you want a lasting effect, you must acknowledge that this is not a one-time deal, but a lifestyle we as humans should embrace. Maintenance of IF that suits your schedule and occasional cyclical EF as part of one's routine actually saves time, money and resources and meal time more meaning during an eating window.

- *Can I recommend this way of life to others?* Yes, you can definitely recommend this way of life to others provided you know the basic dos and don'ts. However, know that no matter how good your intentions are, some people will react very negatively about it and will even humiliate you because. Thus, a word of advice, choose wisely whom you share this knowledge and make sure you are confident enough to answer whatever questions they may throw. But to be safe, why not just recommend reading this book instead? I would really appreciate that. ☺

REFERENCES/SUGGESTED READINGS:

1. https://www.who.int/news-room/fact-sheets/detail/the-top-10-causes-of-death

2. https://siimland.com/everything-about-getting-enough-electrolytes-while-fasting/

3. http://siimland.com/keto-if-fasting/

4. Cahill Jr, G.F., 2006. Fuel metabolism in starvation. *Annu. Rev. Nutr.*, *26*, pp.1-22.

5. Castellini, M.A. and Rea, L.D., 1992. The biochemistry of natural fasting at its limits. *Experientia*, *48*(6), pp.575-582.

6. Izumida, Y., Yahagi, N., Takeuchi, Y., Nishi, M., Shikama, A., Takarada, A., Masuda, Y., Kubota, M., Matsuzaka, T., Nakagawa, Y. and Iizuka, Y., 2013. Glycogen shortage during fasting triggers liver–brain–adipose neurocircuitry to facilitate fat utilization. *Nature communications*, *4*, p.2316.

7. Sarah C. Couch (7 April 2006). "Ask an Expert: Fasting and starvation mode". University of Cincinnati (NetWellness). Archived from the original on 19 July 2011

8. Anton, S.D., Moehl, K., Donahoo, W.T., Marosi, K., Lee, S.A., Mainous III, A.G., Leeuwenburgh, C. and Mattson, M.P., 2018. Flipping the metabolic switch:

understanding and applying the health benefits of fasting. *Obesity*, *26*(2), pp.254-268.

9. https://universityhealthnews.com/daily/nutrition/leptin-foods-answer-always-hungry/

10. Stephens, Gin. Delay: Don´t Deny, Living an Intermittent Fasting Lifestyle

11. Fung, J. The Obesity Code: Unlocking the Secrets of Weight Loss

12. Fung J, Moore J. The Ultimate Guide to Fasting: Heal Your Body Through Intermittent, Alternate Day and Extended Fasting.

13. The Magic Pill at https://www.netflix.com/

14. https://dailyhealthpost.com/fasti
ng-regenerate-immune-
system/?fbclid=IwAR1HlPY1-
_foaza47SphcUCHqxKuPiFAPbO
eW0FR3P2q7Cf9mm02am7ysZA

15. https://www.medicalnewstoday.
com/articles/306638.php 16.

16. https://www.delish.com/food/g2
2617665/celebrities-intermittent-
fasting/

17. https://idmprogram.com/refeedin
g-syndromes-fasting-20/

18. https://www.allaboutfasting.com
/breaking-a-fast.html

APPENDIX A

<u>Minnesota Starvation Experiment</u>

A study in 1944 called the Minnesota Starvation Experiment was done among 36 middle-aged Caucasian men, where caloric restriction was conducted and adjusted so the men can lose 1.1 kilogram per week. The study period was divided into four phases:

1. **Control Period**, wherein they were allowed to eat about 3,200 kcal per day for 12 weeks, and adjusted so the participants will reach their ideal weight for their height in preparation for the next phase.

2. **Semi-Starvation Period**, is a 24-week or 6 months' worth of caloric restriction at 1,560/day. The most important part in here is the type of food that they eat, which is basically carbohydrates (bread, potatoes, turnips, pasta, among others). With calorie deprivation and nutrient-deficient meals, the participants are at their hungriest, very irritable, felt weak and always starving. During this stage, these meal preparations induced depression, hysteria and severe emotional distress from constant mental preoccupation of food, with great anticipation during

their scheduled meal time. They also showed decline in concentration, comprehension and judgment. One participant was even dismissed from the experiment after showing signs of threat to others and his own. Overall, the basal metabolic rate, or the resting energy expenditure also decreased.

3. **Restricted Rehabilitation Period** is the third phase wherein the participants were divided into four groups where they received 400, 800, 1200 or 1600 additional calories from their previous allowance in an aim to know the optimum

amount of calories needed to re-nourish them after losing approximately 25% of their weight. However, even with additional vitamins, participants were not improving especially on the lowest calorie group. Total calorie was adjusted and the researcher concluded that a 4,000 kcal is needed to re-establish their previous health.

4. **Unrestrictive Rehabilitation Period**, wherein for the last 8 weeks, food intake was already unrestricted. However, review of the participants years after the experiment showed psychological impact especially

with food, that they had a hard time adjusting after and were noted to overeat up to 11,000 kcal in a day with fear of having food taken away anytime and be deprived again.

There was no mention on the report on the actual weight changes of the participants after only that it took some time before they returned to the "normal" size. But as to whether what their normal is, we will never know.

The Semi Starvation Period is exactly why the low fat, low calorie diet fad is not sustainable simply because you are battling hunger hormones and decreased metabolism.

This is in contrast with the overwhelming positive effects of intentional, conscious and healthy way of fasting, especially when done on maintenance phase of intermittent fasting. Benefits include improvements on the person's physical as well as emotional well-being, improved psychological status, mental strength and general wellness.

APPENDIX B
Different 20-gram carbohydrates

Different perspectives on how a **20-gram carbohydrates** *will look like*

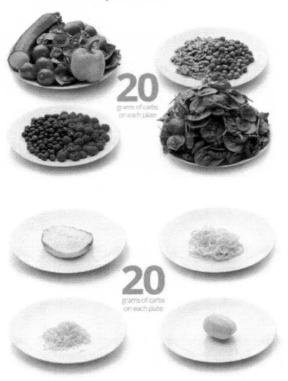

APPENDIX C

Basal Metabolic Index Chart

Underweight | Healthy | Overweight | Obese | Extremely obese

WEIGHT lbs	100	105	110	115	120	125	130	135	140	145	150	155	160	165	170	175	180	185	190	195	200	205	210	215
kgs	46.5	47.7	50.0	52.3	54.5	56.8	59.1	61.4	63.6	65.9	68.2	70.5	72.7	75.0	77.3	79.5	81.8	84.1	86.4	88.6	90.9	93.2	95.5	97.7
HEIGHT in/cm																								
5'0" - 152.4	19	20	21	22	23	24	25	26	27	28	29	30	31	32	33	34	35	36	37	38	39	40	41	42
5'1" - 154.9	18	19	20	21	22	23	24	25	26	27	28	29	30	31	32	33	34	35	36	36	37	38	39	40
5'2" - 157.4	18	19	20	21	22	22	23	24	25	26	27	28	29	30	31	32	33	33	34	35	36	37	38	39
5'3" - 160.0	17	18	19	20	21	22	23	24	24	25	26	27	28	29	30	31	32	32	33	34	35	36	37	38
5'4" - 162.5	17	18	18	19	20	21	22	23	24	24	25	26	27	28	29	30	31	31	32	33	34	35	36	37
5'5" - 165.1	16	17	18	19	20	20	21	22	23	24	25	25	26	27	28	29	30	30	31	32	33	34	35	35
5'6" - 167.6	16	17	17	18	19	20	21	21	22	23	24	25	25	26	27	28	29	29	30	31	32	33	34	34
5'7" - 170.1	15	16	17	18	18	19	20	21	22	22	23	24	25	25	26	27	28	29	29	30	31	32	33	33
5'8" - 172.7	15	16	16	17	18	19	19	20	21	22	22	23	24	25	25	26	27	28	28	29	30	31	32	32
5'9" - 175.2	14	15	16	17	17	18	19	20	20	21	22	22	23	24	25	25	26	27	28	28	29	30	31	31
5'10" - 177.8	14	15	15	16	17	18	18	19	20	20	21	22	23	23	24	25	25	26	27	28	28	29	30	30
5'11" - 180.3	14	14	15	16	16	17	18	18	19	20	21	21	22	23	23	24	25	25	26	27	28	28	29	30
6'0" - 182.8	13	14	14	15	16	17	17	18	19	19	20	21	21	22	23	23	24	25	25	26	27	27	28	29
6'1" - 185.4	13	13	14	15	15	16	17	17	18	19	19	20	21	21	22	23	23	24	25	25	26	27	27	28
6'2" - 187.9	12	13	14	14	15	16	16	17	18	18	19	19	20	21	21	22	23	23	24	25	25	26	27	27
6'3" - 190.5	12	13	13	14	15	15	16	16	17	18	18	19	20	20	21	21	22	23	23	24	25	25	26	26
6'4" - 193.0	12	12	13	14	14	15	15	16	17	17	18	18	19	20	20	21	22	22	23	23	24	25	25	26

APPENDIX D

Sample Intermittent Fasting Schedules

First Meal	Last Meal	Eating Window	Total Fasting
9AM	5PM	8 Hours	16 Hours
10AM	6PM	8 Hours	16 Hours
11AM	7PM	8 Hours	16 Hours
12NN	7PM	8 Hours	16 Hours
12NN	6PM	7 Hours	17 Hours
12NN	5PM	6 Hours	18 Hours
1PM	6PM	5 Hours	19 Hours
1PM	5PM	4 Hours	20 Hours
2PM	6PM	4 Hours	20 Hours
3PM	7PM	4 Hours	20 Hours
3PM	8PM	5 Hours	19 Hours
4PM	9PM	5 Hours	19 Hours

APPENDIX E

Sample Short-term EF Schedules

Type	TIME	8AM	12NN	4PM	6PM	8PM
42H Fast 3x per week	Day 1	Fast	Eat	Eat	Eat	Fast
	Day 2	Fast	Fast	Fast	Fast	Fast
	Day 3	Fast	Eat	Eat	Eat	Fast
	Day 4	Fast	Fast	Fast	Fast	Fast
	Day 5	Fast	Eat	Eat	Eat	Fast
	Day 6	Fast	Fast	Fast	Fast	Fast
	Day 7	Fast	Eat	Eat	Eat	Fast

Type	TIME	8AM	12NN	4PM	6PM	8PM
24H Fast 3x per week	Day 1	Fast	Eat	Eat	Eat	Fast
	Day 2	Fast	Fast	Fast	Eat	Eat
	Day 3	Fast	Eat	Eat	Eat	Fast
	Day 4	Fast	Fast	Fast	Eat	Eat
	Day 5	Fast	Eat	Eat	Eat	Fast
	Day 6	Fast	Fast	Fast	Eat	Eat
	Day 7	Fast	Eat	Eat	Eat	Fast

Type	TIME	8AM	12NN	4PM	6PM	8PM
ADF **or** **36hr** **Fast**	Day 1	Fast	Fast	Fast	Fast	Fast
	Day 2	Eat	Eat	Eat	Eat	Eat
	Day 3	Fast	Fast	Fast	Fast	Fast
	Day 4	Eat	Eat	Eat	Eat	Eat
	Day 5	Fast	Fast	Fast	Fast	Fast
	Day 6	Eat	Eat	Eat	Eat	Eat
	Day 7	Fast	Fast	Fast	Fast	Fast

APPENDIX F

Let's Start This Journey Together

Start by writing down your goals like desired weight, BMI, waist/hips/arm measurements or body fat percentage, or even some "non-scale victory" (NSV) like fitting back to an old *smaller* dress. Trust that you can achieve it. After knowing all the details on fasting and low-carbohydrate diet, you are now ready to design your own routine. If not, let me give you two ways to do it.

The first approach is the fast, jumpstart approach wherein you directly indulge into a minimum of 5 days fasting to ensure that you will be in full ketosis by the time you break your fast. This is how we started in our family. As we are convinced that we can do it, we have each other to support one another. We also choose to have this in a fairly normal week with no extra physically draining tasks. At work, I have informed my workmates that I am in an extended fast and even asked my superior that I will be converting my lunch-break to resting break should I ever feel lightheaded or the need to rest. Surprisingly, that did not come. Except for the feeling of mouth dryness and occasional weakness, we feel as normal as we can be. The weakness was instantly relieved by intake of water with salt and some apple cider vinegar for potassium and sodium. The hunger that happen 2-3x a day persisted but the intensity keeps getting smaller and smaller each day. Whenever there's food temptations, instead of avoiding them, I savor their smell and I convince myself that I know how they taste so well, because I've tasted them many times before and I can eat it any time after, but right at that moment, I am in the most crucial time of making something better out of myself. I am in the process of becoming my best version. I think to myself, "What is one week as compared to a lifetime that I have spent indulging in food with regrets after which led me to a body type I so wanted to improve?", "Or the optimum health and physique that I can achieve from this point onwards?" You may have doubts but remember, there is no shame in trying. The fact that you are open to making good changes with your life starting with your commitment to better health is already commendable in itself.

If at any point you feel tired, you can rest at any time, or stop at any time and start again when you are ready. There was even a time where I have planned for a week-long fast but ended up doing a 24 or 40 hour fast instead simply because I listened to my body. There is no need to rush if you feel you are already endangering yourself. However, should you feel positive about it, you can do the following:

- Day 1 to 3- Clean, water-only fasting, may have salt and apple cider or pure coconut vinegar or (*unsqueezed*) lemon water, green tea and black coffee

- Days 3 to 6 - Continue clean fasting, may take a multivitamin with magnesium if deemed necessary. If it is not enough, you can proceed with *dirty fasting* like having a bulletproof coffee, bone broth and others as previously specified.

- Day 7 - If you can no longer extend it beyond 7 days, slowly break your fast by eating vegetable soup first, and after an hour, eat a proper low carbohydrate meal. Limit your eating window to only 5 hours at maximum. Eat slowly and pleasurably. However, if you feel you can still go another day, you can freely do so.

- Day 8 onwards - you can do 16 or 18 hours daily intermittent fasting
  for weeks doing strictly a low carb diet.

- Day 21 - you may repeat another cycle of extended fast or continue your IF or engage on OMAD until you reach your desired goal. Just trust the process, because slowly yet surely, you will get there even with or without exercise.

The second approach are mostly followed by my friends whom I don't see on a day to day basis, to which the daily encouragement and monitoring is somewhat limited as compared to my family that I live with.

If you have never heard of IF, and are apprehensive on how this is going to work out, you can start by slowly extending your overnight fast. As explained earlier, make it into a goal to have at least 16 hours of fasting daily. You can have 1 light meal to open your window, have a proper meal in between and another light meal to close it. Or you can have two proper meals upon opening and another one before closing your *"eating window"*, with nothing but coffee, tea or water in between the two meals. Follow this routine for at least two months and see the difference yourself. Some may not have significant weight loss per se, but people will start to notice how your face and body slowly improves in shape, including clearer skin, more toned structure and lighter appearance. Common non-scale benefits include decreased inflammation, joint pains and even allergies. The moment you graduate from a month of IF, you can level up to OMAD and even try extended fasting slowly in time.

I know it is much easier if you have a support group as you decide to embark in this journey, but you have to accept the fact that there is a possibility that you might be going through this alone, and you have to persist despite the circumstances. You will be the one that will rip the benefits after all. Right now, we have a support (closed) group in Facebook where you are most welcome to join. Just look for the group named **"Perfect At Last Support Group"**. You can also join various international support groups in Facebook where people openly support each other's journey.

Always be psychologically prepared that sometimes, the people closest to you will be the ones discouraging or tempting you to break your fast or eat the sugary snacks you are doing your best to resist. Know your goals and know yourself. Make these two months a test of self-love and a beginning of self-care your body has been craving for.

In the beginning, I find it beneficial that I cleaned out my pantry first. I gave away all the simple sugars, biscuits and juices that I have. Then, I bought a week supply of cabbage and eggs as my staple. I downloaded the app **LIF**E for fasting to keep track of my daily fast (*Join me and many others. Just look for the fasting circle named Limitless* ♥). I placed the red list and green list on the dining table.

I made a daily routine for going to work early and getting myself busy during the day. As a result, I sleep regularly earlier than I used to. During the weekends or during idle times when I cannot help but think about food, I fill up my time watching really binge-worthy shows or some *YouTube* videos on the benefits of fasting and related videos like "how to fast successfully". Aside from enriching my knowledge, it successfully helped me to overcome one cycle of almost 11 days, one cycle of 7 days and one cycle of 5 days water fasting, one cycle of 5 and 3 days of dirty fasting and countless 24-50 hour fasts in 3 months' time with a total of 22 pounds sustained weight loss without exercise.

I was a sugar and food addict. *Coke* has been like water. And I was raised in an environment where the definition of fullness is when you can no longer breathe deeply or sit straight. I used to eat very quickly and the only parts I love eating in cakes are the frosting. But now, I am far from where I used to be. And I feel like I already got my share of carb indulgence one is expected to have in a lifetime that I must now embark on this low-carbohydrate lifestyle forever. But to be honest, I know that is impossible. Just now, I ate 6 slices of toasted chiffon cake.

And since that is mostly sugar, I will extend my fast to 36 hours, so I make sure the glucose and glycogen I chose to eat today will be metabolized into the energy that I will need for the succeeding days. See? This is not so bad. Sweets are part of our natural food list. However, you must recognize that sweets naturally come from seasonal fruits or when the hunters stumble upon a beehive once in a while. Thus, if you want to be strict about it, you can have sweets with the frequency similar to that of a seasoned fruit or the chance of finding honey in the wild. But realistically speaking, sweets are already part of our modern day and varieties of fruits are practically available all year round. You can have it but timing is the key. So long as you strike a balance between regular eating patterns, occasional feast and planned fast, you can achieve the health and physique our hunter-gatherer ancestors used to have.

I will leave the decision to you on how you will go about it. You can start strong with extended fast and maintain on OMAD and pure LCHF diet - what I consider to be the most effective and the most efficient. Or you can slowly ease in with increasing IF and OMAD while eating whatever you can, especially incorporating sugars during your window. Again, there is no such thing as perfection that is uniform for everyone, but there is always something that is perfect for you, and time is in your hands in order for you to learn it little by little each day. Feel free to experiment and see for yourself what works for you and the life you plan to have.

Again, add me on Facebook, follow me *Instagram* or send me an email and I'd be more than willing to help as soon as time allows. ☺

APPENDIX G
List and Recipe of Easy, Affordable

Low Carb, High Fiber Alternatives

- **Buttered Bland Greens** - Use finely chopped cabbage, broccoli and/or cauliflower and sauté it in butter. You can mix it with whatever food you fancy on the above green list. The more common they are, the better your compliance will be. The longer you cook them, the lesser they taste, thus the more palatable they become. However, if you are used to their raw taste, you can eat them just as soon as the butter melts to maximize intake of the nutrients.

- **High Fiber Omelets** - you can use whole eggs or just the white egg and cook the yolk separately and serve as a different side dish. For a single full serving, you can beat 1-2 eggs, and add 2-4 cups of chopped greens and that's it to be paired with your main fatty meat. An alternative would be 4 tablespoons of whole oats, or 2 tablespoon of ground flaxseed meal or *psyllium* husk powder. You can add cheese, cream cheese, coconut flour or almond flour, whatever is available and depending on your preferred consistency. This is very filling and a perfect match to any meat.

- **Fresh salads** - lettuce, finely chopped cabbage and bell peppers, cucumber, tomato, all mixed together or alone, with real mayo, some salt and a teaspoon of vinegar is just one of our table staples. These are very easy to buy and to prepare without the need for cooking! Olive oil is the best oil to use for raw meals.

- **Noodles and Pasta without the Carbs** - Whether it's a chicken or beef soup, or red or white pasta dish, just cook it as but replace the noodles and pasta with steamed cauliflower or fine strips of vegetables. With these, you won't be missing any of them anymore. Cook in pure coconut cooking oil or butter or lard.

These are just samples and my favorite ones because they are very cheap, doesn't get spoil easily, delicious and very easy to prepare. The more fiber-rich foods you can tolerate, the raw, the better. You can put in other low-carb favorites and create your own.

APPENDIX H

Low Carbohydrate Dessert

There are thousands of easy low carb desserts available online, but two of my favorites are as follows:

1. **Dark Chocolate** - Just mix 1 cup of 100% pure cocoa, 250gms of cream cheese and 5 tablespoon of Monk fruit sweetener and pour into chocolate bar molds or even small cupcake cups. If you add 1 cup of heavy cream, it will be converted into a chocolate pudding. Chill and serve.

1. **Avocado Ice Cream** - Puree 4 cups of sliced avocado, add 250gms heavy cream and 4 tablespoon Monk fruit sweetener or stevia counterpart. Chill and serve.

There are hundreds more, but to cure a sweet tooth and silence the chocolate monster within, a bite of these treats surely fits.

APPENDIX I

Ketogenic Cooking and Baking

For those who are fond of baking, there are a lot of common ketogenic counterparts. Found in the internet. Once you've mastered the art of having low carbohydrate dishes, you can maximize the benefit by converting it into a ketogenic meal where those low-carb alternative be paired with a healthy fatty main course. Examples would include pork, salmon, lamb and many more. Refer to the green list for the foods you can eat and the red list as the items you should avoid.

Although calorie counting is not really recommended, but by proportion, 60-75% of your energy foods must come from fats, 25-30% from proteins and 5% from carbs. That 5% of carbs are usually less than 20 grams per day. Start reading labels if you buy processed foods and avoid those with carbohydrate or sugar content more than 1 gram per serving, unless it's the only thing you will consume for the day.

Closing Message

To you,

By now, I hope you are done reading the whole book. I know there may still be doubts within you especially with the uncertainty whether you can do it or not. I understand it is a lot to take in. But if there is a minimum take home message that I want everyone to have, it's these:

- *Fasting is a natural process.*

- *It is okay not to eat all the time.*

- *Unintentional skipped meals should not be a cause of worry, but be celebrated.*

- *If EF is too much or unnecessary for you, then doing IF for as long as you can is the next best step.*

- *Ketogenic diet, to some extent, biochemically mimics the effect of fasting through ketosis in a slower pace.*

- *Can't let go of carbs? Compensate by fasting.*

- *Can't afford an extended fast? Compensate by eating LCHF foods.*

- *Want to have the best results the fastest way? Do both!*

- *When asked why you fast, just answer "It's because I can", with confidence.*

- *Lastly, if you are asked by anybody what you are doing, in a limited time and avenue to explain things completely, then I humbly suggest for you to avoid talking about "fasting". Because they will probably just raise an eyebrow and close their minds even before you say another word. Instead, you can show them the results and wait until they are truly interested and have a proper time and place to talk about it substantially and completely. It is the main reason why fasting is not mentioned in the cover of the book, in hope that in the end, even a close-minded reader will have the acceptance that it is a natural part of human existence, whether or not he/she chooses to practice such.*

If you think somebody else you care about can benefit from this book, pay it forward by sharing it with them or giving one as a gift.

Thank you very much for hearing me all these times. Whatever path you choose, I hope it is the one directed towards self-love and achieving your best version yet.

I wish you all the best in this journey.

Yours,

Grace

Copyright

This copy is intended for

_____.

Illegal distribution, printing or production of this book is
strictly prohibited.

This book is under copyright protection and shall not be
reproduced in any form without the consent of the
author.

If you wish to share a copy, kindly refer to
www.healthandwellnessforless.info
Or email me at
jgcrojomd@healthandwellnessforless.info

Perfect At Last Book Series
All rights reserved.

Josephine Grace Chua Rojo
Copyright 2019

ISBN: 9781691732487
Lulu Publishing

www.healthandwellnessforless.info

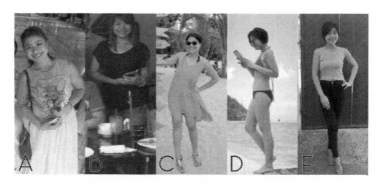

Photos A - B were taken in 2017. C was in late
2018. D in March 2019, E taken in June 2019

Made in the USA
Middletown, DE
21 February 2022

61600656R00191